Head, Neck, and Dental Anatomy

Third Edition

MARJORIE J. SHORT, R.D.H., B.S., M.S.

Formerly a Professor at
Middlesex Community College, Lowell, MA

This edition revised by the author of the
Head and Neck Anatomy Section
DEBORAH LEVIN-GOLDSTEIN, R.D.H., B.S., M.S.
Professor, Dental Hygiene
Northampton Community College, Bethlehem, PA

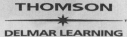
THOMSON

DELMAR LEARNING

Australia Canada Mexico Singapore Spain United Kingdom United States

THOMSON

DELMAR LEARNING

Head, Neck, and Dental Anatomy, Third Edition
by Marjorie J. Short and Deborah Levin-Goldstein

Executive Director, Health Care Business Unit:
William Brottmiller

Executive Editor:
Cathy L. Esperti

Acquisitions Editor:
Maureen Rosener

Editorial Assistant:
Matthew Thouin

Executive Marketing Manager:
Dawn F. Gerrain

Channel Manager:
Jennifer McAvey

Production Editor:
Mary Colleen Liburdi

Library of Congress Cataloging-in-Publication Data

Short, Marjorie J., 1935–
   Head, neck, and dental anatomy / Marjorie J. Short ; this edition revised by the author of the head and neck anatomy section, Deborah Levin-Goldstein.—3rd ed.
      p. ; cm.
   Includes bibliographical references and index.
   ISBN: 0-7668-1889-6
   1. Head—Anatomy. 2. Neck—Anatomy. 3. Mouth—Anatomy. 4. Teeth—Anatomy. I. Levin-Goldstein, Deborah. II. Title.
   [DNLM: 1. Tooth—anatomy & histology. 2. Head—anatomy & histology. 3. Neck—anatomy & histology. WU 101-S559e 2002]
QM535 .S48 2002
611'.91—dc21
                              2002067516

NOTICE TO THE READER

Preface

This textbook is written for dental assisting students as an introduction to the study of anatomy of the teeth, head and neck. The Instructor's Manual is a new feature for the third edition. It combines review questions, clinical and laboratory applications and case studies into one place for ease in teaching.

SPECIAL FEATURES

This book has several special features that enhance its usefulness to both the teacher and student.

- *Outstanding Art Program.* This book has been extensively revised to include clear drawings of the teeth and precise illustrations of head anatomy.
- *Tooth Identification Charts.* The most important features of each tooth are detailed in a brief, concise chart. These charts are an excellent study guide for students.
- *The Instructor's Manual.* This Manual is a wonderful resource for the didactic teacher.
- *In-text Student Aids.* Objectives, Summaries, and Review Questions alert students to the most important concepts in each chapter, and help them recall and test their knowledge.

- *Clinical Consideration*. Particular attention is directed to root anatomy of each tooth, identifying structures that will be detected by dental assistants during tooth examination and exploration.
- *Clinical Applications*. Clinical laboratory exercises are included to emphasize the importance of form to function. It is often easier to remember details by observing them directly as they would be seen from a clinical point of view. This helps to relate dental anatomy to the use of instruments, preventive care, or restorative dentistry.

ACKNOWLEDGMENTS

This textbook would not be possible without the support of my husband, Dr. Howard M. Goldstein, and my son, Mark. I would like to extend my thanks and love to them.

Reviewer List

Lana Barnett-Edwards, DMD
Dental Assisting / Dental Hygiene
Department
Lewis & Clark Community College
Godfrey, IL

Eugenia B. Bearden, RDH., M.Ed.
Clayton College and State University
Morrow, GA

Cheryl Chinn, BS, MA, RDH
Dental Hygiene Department
Sacramento City College
Sacramento, CA

Linda Kay Hughes, RDA, NRDA
Excelle Medical and Dental College
San Diego, CA

Gail Kilpatrick, CDA, BS
Dental Assisting Program
Warren Technical Center
Golden, CO

Rebecca Matney, CDA, RDA
Dental Assisting Department
Vatterott College
Springfield, MO

Debbie M. Reynon, CDA, RDA, AA, AS
Santa Cruz County Office of Education
Dental Assisting Program
Santa Cruz, CA

Jeanette Shahboz, CDA
Miami-Dade County Public School
Miami, FL

Donna Jeanne Wedell, RDA, CDA
Dental Assisting Department
Cerritos College, Norwalk, CA
Orange Coast College, Costa Mesa, CA

Contents

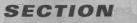

I

Introduction to the Oral Cavity

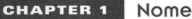

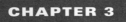

Nomenclature

KEY TERMS

Dentition

Deciduous

Permanent

Exfoliate

Mixed dentition

Succedaneous

Diphyodonts

Polyphyodonts

Heterodonts

Mastication

Anterior

Posterior

Eruption

Active eruption

Passive eruption

Attrition

Abrasion

The Dentition
The Names and Functions of the Teeth
The Arrangement of the Teeth
The Eruption Sequence

OBJECTIVES

- Identify, by name, the two dental arches, the permanent teeth, the deciduous teeth, and anterior and posterior teeth.
- Name the teeth in the order in which they are positioned in the dental arch, the function of each type of tooth, and the eruption sequence of deciduous and permanent teeth.
- Define the terms noted in boldface.
- Complete the worksheet at the end of the chapter.
- Perform the clinical applications at the end of the chapter.

THE DENTITION

Teeth are arranged in the jaws to form two dental arches. Each arch is named to correspond with the bone from which it is composed. The maxilla forms the maxillary or upper arch; the mandible forms the mandibular or lower arch. Together, the two arches make up one **dentition**, or set of teeth (Figure 1-1). During the life span, each person normally will have two dentitions, the **primary (deciduous)** and the **permanent**.

The Primary (Deciduous) Dentition

The first or primary set of teeth, the deciduous dentition, begins to emerge into the mouth between 6 and 8 months of age. Teeth continue to erupt periodically, following a developmental schedule, until 20 teeth, 10 maxillary and 10 mandibular, have erupted by the age of 2 $1/2$–3 years. These 20 deciduous teeth are small, but they fulfill the needs of a child. As the child grows, the deciduous teeth eventually **exfoliate**, or shed, and are replaced by permanent teeth. When all the permanent teeth have erupted, by the ages of 17 through 21, the permanent dentition is complete (Figure 1-1).

The Permanent Dentition

There are 32 permanent teeth, 16 maxillary and 16 mandibular. Until the child is 5 years old, only deciduous teeth are present in the mouth. Between 5 and 6 years of age, the first permanent tooth, the mandibular first molar,

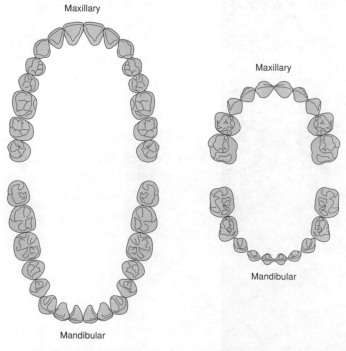

FIGURE 1–1
(A) Maxillary and mandibular dentition of an adult (permanent dentition).
(B) Maxillary and mandibular dentition of a child (primary dentition).

(A) Permanent dentition   **(B) Primary (deciduous) dentition**

erupts posterior to the last deciduous molar. No deciduous tooth has exfoliated to provide space for this permanent tooth; however, the mandible has increased in length so that there is now space for an additional tooth. Permanent molars do not replace or succeed deciduous teeth (Figure 1-1).

Shortly after the permanent first molars erupt, deciduous incisors, the front teeth, begin to exfoliate. This occurs as a result of a physiologic process that causes their roots to resorb as the permanent teeth form in the bone directly beneath them. Eventually, every deciduous tooth should exfoliate and be succeeded by a permanent tooth.

Between the ages of 5 and 12, some deciduous and some permanent teeth are present in the mouth at the same time; this is referred to as a **mixed dentition**. Permanent teeth that replace or succeed deciduous teeth are called **succedaneous** teeth and include incisors, canines, and premolars. Permanent molars are not succedaneous teeth because they do not replace deciduous teeth.

Because human beings have two successive sets of teeth during their lives (a deciduous and a permanent dentition), they are considered **diphyodonts**. Having several sets of teeth throughout life, as certain reptiles do, would make the species **polyphyodonts**.

THE NAMES AND FUNCTIONS OF THE TEETH

Each dentition includes several types of teeth shaped to perform specific functions. People are **heterodonts** because they have different types of teeth called incisors, canines, premolars, and molars. The types of teeth in the maxillary arch are the same as those in the mandibular arch. When an imaginary midline is drawn to divide the arches into a right and left quadrant, the teeth in the right quadrant are the same as those in the left quadrant.

The Permanent Teeth

As mentioned, the permanent dentition has 32 teeth, 16 maxillary and 16 mandibular (see Figure 1-2).

Types of Teeth	Number on each arch
Incisors are the four front teeth and have sharp biting edges for incising, or cutting food. The two in the middle of the arch are central incisors; those on each side are lateral incisors.	4
Canines, also called cuspids, are the corner teeth and have one pointed cusp used to hold and tear food.	2
Premolars, also called bicuspids, are posterior teeth having two major cusps adapted to crush and tear food. Premolars are named by the sequence in the arch from front to back as "first premolar" and "second premolar."	4
Molars are broad back teeth having several cusps adapted to chew, crush, and grind food. They, too, are named by their sequence from the front to the back of the arch as "first molar," "second molar," and "third molar."	6
	16 total per arch

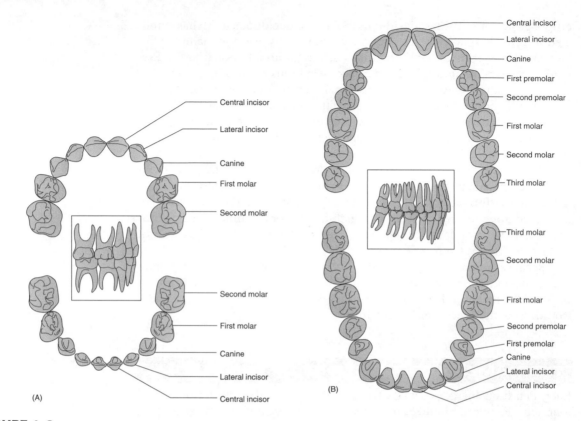

FIGURE 1–2

(A) The primary dentition identifying each tooth by name. (B) The permanent dentition identifying each tooth by name.

Each tooth performs its individual function in the process of mastication, or chewing. By working together, the teeth prepare food for swallowing and digestion.

The Primary (Deciduous) Teeth

The deciduous dentition has 20 teeth, 10 maxillary, and 10 mandibular. They are smaller but similar in shape and function to the permanent teeth. They are as follows:

Number on each arch	Types of Teeth
4	*Incisors*—two central and two lateral
2	*Canines*—one in each corner of the arch
4	*Molars*—two first molars, two second molars
10 total per arch	

Each deciduous tooth is eventually replaced by a permanent tooth. Note, however, that there are no primary premolars. Primary molars are succeeded by permanent premolars. Permanent molars erupt posterior to the primary molars without replacing any primary molars. As mentioned, permanent molars are not succedaneous teeth (Figure 1-2).

THE ARRANGEMENT OF THE TEETH

Figure 1-2 shows the arrangement of the permanent teeth in the dental arches. The **anterior** teeth are those in the front of the mouth and include incisors and canines. **Posterior** teeth, those in the back of the mouth, include premolars and molars.

Tooth Description

To identify a tooth correctly, note that it is designated not only by its name and arch but also by the quadrant in which it is located. Each quadrant is specified according to the patient's right or left side. To completely identify a tooth, provide information in the following sequence:

	DENTITION	ARCH	QUADRANT	TOOTH
Example	Permanent	Mandibular	Right	Central Incisor

THE ERUPTION SEQUENCE

Although teeth begin to form in utero, eruptions occur at approximately 6–8 months of age. **Eruption** dates vary from person to person by a few months, just as the individual growth rate varies. Table 1-1 lists the eruption

TABLE 1–1 ERUPTION AND EXFOLIATION DATES FOR PRIMARY TEETH			
Tooth	**Eruption Date**	**Exfoliation Date**	**Maxillary Order**
Central incisor	6–10 months	6–7 years	#1
Lateral incisor	9–12 months	7–8 years	#2
Canine	16–22 months	10–12 years	#4
First molar	12–18 months	9–11 years	#3
Second molar	24–32 months	10–12 years	#5
			Mandibular Order
Central incisor	6–10 months	6–7 years	#1
Lateral incisor	7–10 months	7–8 years	#2
Canine	16–22 months	9–12 years	#4
First molar	12–18 months	9–11 years	#3
Second molar	20–32 months	10–12 years	#5

sequence for **primary teeth**. Note that mandibular teeth generally precede maxillary teeth in eruption.

By the age of $2\frac{1}{2}$–3 years, all deciduous teeth have erupted; at about 6 years, the permanent teeth start to erupt. Refer to Figure 1-3 for the growth pattern of the teeth. A chronology of this growth pattern is given in Appendix A.

The first molars are the first permanent teeth to emerge into the mouth. They erupt posterior to the deciduous second molar without replacing any deciduous teeth. The eruption sequence of the permanent dentition is shown in Table 1-2.

The initial eruption period, called **active eruption**, continues until the crown is almost completely exposed and the tooth is in its proper align-

TABLE 1–2   ERUPTION DATES FOR PERMANENT TEETH

Tooth	Eruption Date	Order of Eruption (Maxillary)
Central incisor	7–8 years	#2
Lateral incisor	8–9 years	#3
Canine	11–12 years	#6
First premolar	10–11 years	#4
Second premolar	11–12 years	#5
First molar	6–7 years	#1
Second molar	12–13 years	#7
Third molar	17–21 years	#8
		Order of Eruption (Mandibular)
Central incisor	6–7 years	#2
Lateral incisor	7–8 years	#3
Cuspid	9–10 years	#4
First premolar	10–11 years	#5
Second premolar	11–12 years	#6
First molar	6–7 years	#1
Second molar	11–13 years	#7
Third molar	17–21 years	#8

ment. In later life, the "gums," or gingival line, may recede, exposing more of the tooth. This process is referred to as **passive eruption**.

Development of Human Dentition

Prenatal	Infancy	Early Childhood

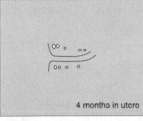

4 months in utero

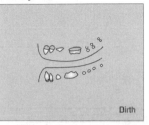

Birth

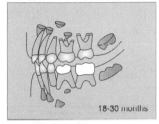

18-30 months

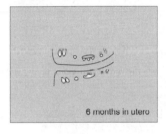

6 months in utero

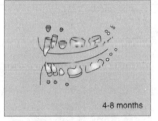

4-8 months

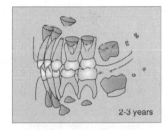

2-3 years

 Primary Dentition

 Permanent Dentition

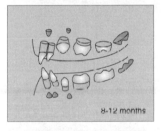

8-12 months

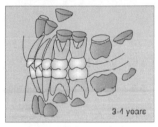

3-4 years

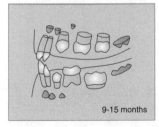

9-15 months

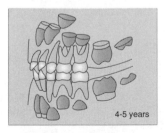

4-5 years

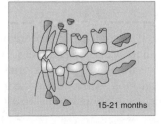

15-21 months

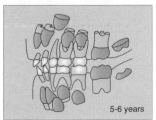

5-6 years

FIGURE 1–3
Development of the Human Dentition

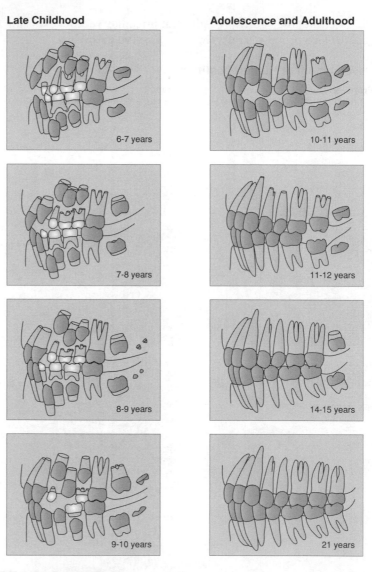

FIGURE 1–3, Continued
Stages of Tooth Eruption
Copyright by the American Dental Association. Reprinted with permission, 2002.

Continual use of the teeth throughout life can cause a slight wearing away of the biting and/or chewing surfaces and, hence, a decrease in the height of the tooth. This wearing away is called **attrition**. Grinding of the teeth (bruxism) also causes attrition. **Abrasion** of the tooth surfaces can be caused by mechanical wear such as continual biting on an object or brushing too vigorously.

SUMMARY

During a person's life span there will be two sets of teeth. The first set, the primary or deciduous dentition, consists of 20 teeth. It eventually exfoliates and is replaced by the permanent dentition, which has 32 teeth.

Each dentition has several types of teeth shaped to perform specific functions; they work in conjunction with one another to prepare the food for digestion.

Deciduous teeth begin to emerge during the sixth month of infancy, but they are not completely erupted as a full dentition until the third year of life. Permanent teeth begin to emerge between 5 and 6 years of age, and all but the third molars have usually erupted by the twelfth year. Permanent teeth are expected to last a lifetime.

WORKSHEET

A. Define the following words.

Active eruption _____

Anterior_____

Attrition_____

Deciduous teeth _____

Dentition _____

Diphyodont _____

Exfoliate _____

Heterodont _____

Mastication _____

Passive Eruption_____

Polyphyodont _____

Posterior _____

Succedaneous_____

B. Clinical Applications

A dental mouth mirror is required for the following exercises. Before completing them, observe the shapes of the teeth, noticing how they differ. Have your patient open and close the teeth, noticing the manner in which they interdigitate.

1. Describe the shapes of the teeth and relate this to their specific function.

   a. incisors

   b. canines

   c. premolars

   d. molars

2. Observe the biting edges and chewing surfaces. Record those teeth that have attrition and the reason you feel this occurred.

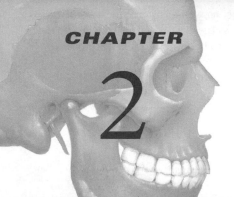

Structures of the Oral Cavity

Related Terminology
The Oral Cavity
Structures External to the Oral Cavity
Structures of the Oral Vestibule
Structures of the Oral Cavity Proper

OBJECTIVES

- Identify two areas of the oral cavity, the boundaries of the oral vestibule, and the boundaries of the oral cavity proper.
- Describe each structure of the oral cavity as to location, color, size, and/or shape.
- Define the terms noted in boldface.
- Complete the worksheet at the end of the chapter.
- Perform the clinical applications at the end of the chapter.

RELATED TERMINOLOGY

The names of many oral cavity structures, as well as associated and descriptive terms, are derived from Latin words. As these words appear over and over again throughout the readings, it is helpful to become familiar with them.

Alba	white
Bucca	cheek
Buccal	relating to the cheek
Fornix	arch
Frenum	folds of tissue
Labia	lip
Labial	relating to the lip
Linea	line
Lingual	relating to the tongue
Mental	relating to the chin
Nasal	relating to the nose
Naso	nose
Oral	relating to the mouth
Plica	fold (of tissue)
Raphe	a seam (of tissue)
Sub	under

THE ORAL CAVITY

The term **oral cavity** is used when referring to the inner portion of the mouth. The oral cavity extends from the anterior opening at the lips to the oro-pharynx, or throat posteriorly. The palate, or roof of the mouth, is the superior, or upper, border; and the tongue, along with the musculature beneath it, defines the inferior or lower boundary.

The soft, moist tissue called the *mucous membrane* lines the oral cavity. In the mouth, the mucous membrane is referred to as the **oral mucosa**. The oral mucosa is pink and occurs in various degrees of thickness. Although not as strong or as thick as skin, it acts as a protective covering for the oral cavity. In some areas the oral mucosa is firmly attached, as on the gingiva and hard palate. In other areas, such as the cheek, it is much looser. There are three types of oral mucosa, each classified according to function and location:

1. *Masticatory mucosa* covers areas subject to stress, such as gingival tissue and the hard palate.
2. *Specialized mucosa* covers the area that has the specific function of taste on the dorsum of the tongue.
3. *Lining mucosa* covers all other areas of the oral cavity, such as the inner surfaces of the lips and cheeks and the floor and roof of the mouth.

Divisions

The oral cavity is divided into two sections, the oral vestibule and the oral cavity proper. The **oral vestibule** is the area between the inner lips, or labial mucosa, and cheeks (**buccal** mucosa) and the front (facial) surfaces of the teeth. The *oral cavity proper* extends from the inner (lingual) surfaces of the teeth to the oro-pharynx.

Functions

Chewing of food, or mastication, is the most obvious function of the oral cavity. As chewing occurs, food is moistened with saliva, preparing it for swallowing (deglutition) and digestion. The tongue is the taste organ for food and assists the cheek and lip muscles with movement of food around the oral cavity. In addition to these functions, the oral cavity provides an air passage and assists the tongue with speech.

STRUCTURES EXTERNAL TO THE ORAL CAVITY

The structures of the lips, cheeks, and related areas of the face are closely associated with the oral cavity because they assist with its effective function-ing (Figure 2-1). These outer structures are made up of muscles that aid in opening and closing the lips, and compressing food against as well as mov-ing it away from the teeth. They include:

> **Labial commissure**: the closure line of the lips
> **Philtrum**: shallow depression extending from the area below the middle of the nose to the center of the upper lip
> **Vermilion zone**: the pink border of the lips (thinly keratinized epithelium)
> **Naso-labial groove**: a shallow depression extending from the cor-ner of the nose (ala) to the corner of the lips
> **Labio-mental groove**: a shallow linear depression between the center of the lower lip and the chin
> **Labial tubercle**: a small projection in the middle of the upper lip that may enlarge or thicken

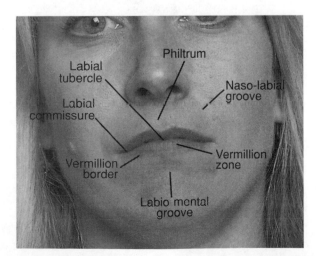

FIGURE 2-1
Landmarks of the face

STRUCTURES OF THE ORAL VESTIBULE

Although the oral vestibule is a small antechamber, it contains several structures that should be recognized (Figure 2-2 and Figure 2-3).

Labial **frenum**: an elevated fold of soft mucous tissue extending from the alveolar mucosa of the two central incisors to the labial mucosa. (A superior frenum exists in the maxillary area; an inferior frenum is located in the mandibular area.) (See Figure 2-3.)

Buccal **frenum**: an elevated fold of soft tissue extending from the alveolar mucosa above the canine or premolar to the buccal mucosa. (See Figure 2-3.)

Maxillary tuberosity: a small, rounded extension of bone, covered with soft tissue, posterior to the last maxillary tooth.

Retromolar area: a triangular area of bone, covered with soft tissue, posterior to the last mandibular tooth.

Stensen's papilla: a small, raised flap of soft tissue on the buccal mucosa opposite the maxillary molar. (It is often marked with a tiny red dot, which is the opening to the parotid or Stensen's salivary gland.)

Linea alba: a raised, white horizontal extension of soft tissue along the buccal mucosa at the occlusal line. (The literal translation of these words is "white line." The linea alba is not present in all mouths.)

Gingiva: pink, stippled mucosa surrounding the necks of the teeth and covering the bone in which the teeth are anchored.

Fordyce granules: small, yellow spots on the buccal mucosa and inner lip. They are sebaceous glands and have no clinical significance.

Anterior tonsillar pillar: folds of tissue that extend horizontally from the uvula to the base of the tongue.

Posterior tonsillar: a set of arches of tissue set farther back in the throat than the anterior tonsillar pillar.

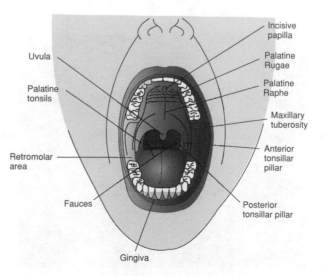

FIGURE 2-2

Landmarks of the palate and oral pharynx area

STRUCTURES OF THE ORAL CAVITY PROPER

Roof of the Mouth

When the mouth is wide open, it is possible to observe all the structures of the oral cavity proper. The following structures are located on the roof of the mouth (see Figure 2-3):

Palate: the concave surface that is known as the roof of the mouth and is divided into the hard and soft palate.

Hard palate: the bony anterior two-thirds of the palate that is covered with mucosa.

Soft palate: the posterior third of the palate, made up of muscular fibers covered with mucosa. (It is a deeper color pink than the hard palate because of its highly vascular composition.)

Palatine torus: a bony prominence of varied size located at the midline of the hard palate. (It is a nonpathologic excess of bone covered with mucosa and only is present in about 20 percent of the population.)

Incisive papilla: a small, raised, rounded structure of soft tissue at the anterior midline of the hard palate. (It is directly behind the two maxillary central incisors and covers and protects the incisive foramen, an opening in the bone directly beneath it through which nerves and blood vessels travel.)

Palatine raphe: a junction of soft tissue extending vertically along the entire midline of the hard palate. Also known as the median palatine raphe.

Palatine rugae: paired raised, palatine folds of soft tissue on the anterior portion of the hard palate. The rugae extend horizontally from the raphe and prevent food from adhering to the palate.

Fovea palatinus: two small indentations, one on either side of the raphe, located at the junction of the hard and soft palate. (These are remnants of minor salivary glands. Their only value is as the terminal demarcation in the fabrication of the maxillary denture.)

Uvula: a downward projection of the soft palate made up of connective tissue, muscles, and glands.

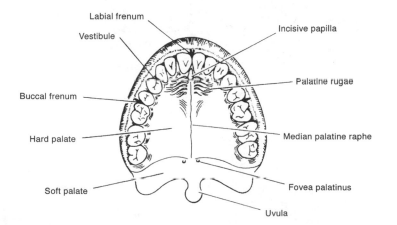

FIGURE 2-3
Structures of the hard and soft palates

Fauces

The following structures are located at the posterior portion of the oral cavity and form the pillars of fauces, the arch or entryway that joins the oral cavity with the pharynx.

> **Oro-pharynx**: the area of the oral cavity that joins it with the throat or pharynx. (On either side are the arches of muscular tissue called the pillars of fauces.)
>
> **Glossopharyngeal muscle**: the anterior pillar of fauces extending from the outer surface of the palate to the tongue.
>
> **Palatopharyngeal muscle**: the posterior pillar of fauces extending from the pharynx to the palate.
>
> **Palatine tonsils**: masses of lymphoid tissue located between the anterior and posterior pillars of fauces.

Tongue

The tongue is a muscular structure covered with oral mucosa. The anterior two-thirds of the tongue is referred to as the body; the posterior third is the base of the tongue. The following structures are located on the *dorsum* of the tongue, as shown in Figure 2-4.

> **Median sulcus**: a shallow groove extending along the midline of the tongue, ending in a slight depression called the foramen caecum.

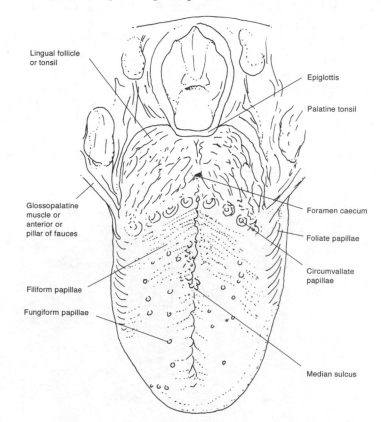

Lingual follicle or tonsil

Epiglottis

Palatine tonsil

Glossopalatine muscle or anterior or pillar of fauces

Foramen caecum

Foliate papillae

Circumvallate papillae

Filiform papillae

Fungiform papillae

Median sulcus

FIGURE 2-4

Structures on the tongue

Foramen caecum: a "V"-shaped terminal sulcus at the posterior area of the median sulcus. It is considered the junction of the oral and pharyngeal sections of the tongue.

There are numerous *papillae* on the dorsum of the tongue:

Circumvallate form a "V" shape and are anterior to the foramen caecum. They vary from 8 to 10 in number and are the largest of the papillae.

Fungiform are located on the sides and apex of the tongue, although they can appear on other portions as well. These are broad, round, red toadstool-shaped papillae.

Filiform are abundantly located on the anterior two-thirds of the tongue. These long, thin, more flexible papillae are greyish in color.

Foliate are located on the lateral surfaces of the posterior third of the tongue. There are 3–5 (or more) of these large raised papillae on each side.

The tongue functions as the main organ of taste and is an important adjunct of speech. It also assists in mastication by rolling and kneading the food against the teeth and hard palate, and in deglutition by pushing the food backward into the oro-pharynx.

Taste buds are located in the papillae of the tongue and are stimulated when food is dissolved. The four primary taste sensations are bitter, sweet, salty, and sour (acid).

PAPILLAE	TASTE
Circumvallate	bitter
Fungiform	sweet, sour, salty
Foliate	sour
Filiform	rarely have taste buds

The base of the tongue is attached. It is continuous with the oral portion, extending downward toward the epiglottis. The lingual tonsils (or lingual follicles), located on the sides of the posterior median line, are nodular masses of lymphoid follicles.

The following structures are located on the floor of the oral cavity. In order for these structures to be observed, the tongue must be raised, as shown in Figure 2-5.

Lingual frenum: an elevated fold of soft tissue located on the floor of the mouth at the midline. It extends from the tissue below the central incisors to the undersurface of the tongue.

Sublingual caruncles: round, elevated sections of soft tissue on either side of the lingual frenum, directly behind the central incisors on the floor of the mouth. Within the caruncles are duct openings to the sublingual (Bartholin's) and submandibular (Wharton's) salivary glands.

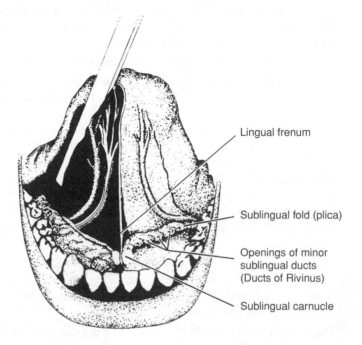

Lingual frenum

Sublingual fold (plica)

Openings of minor sublingual ducts (Ducts of Rivinus)

Sublingual carnucle

FIGURE 2-5
Structures on the floor of the mouth

Sublingual fold: an elevated fold of soft tissue extending, medially, along the floor of the mouth toward the tongue. This fold contains the opening to salivary glands called the *Ducts of Rivinus*.
Mandibular tori: an overgrowth of bone occurring bilaterally on the internal borders of the mandible. As with the maxillary torus, this overgrowth is nonpathologic and occurs in only 8 percent of the population.

SUMMARY

The structures external to the oral cavity include the lips, cheeks, and related areas of the face that assist the oral cavity in functioning effectively.

The entire oral cavity, or mouth, is lined with a soft, moist covering called the *oral mucosa*. This lining has different degrees of consistency that enhance and protect oral structures such as the tongue and hard palate.

The oral cavity is divided into two sections: the oral vestibule and the oral cavity proper, each with its associated structures. It is important to be familiar with the complete anatomy of the oral structures as well as with the terminology necessary for differentiating normal from abnormal.

WORKSHEET

A. *Define the following words.*

Buccal _____

Sub_____

Frenum _____

Labial _____

Lingual _____

Mental _____

Nasal _____

Plica _____

Raphe _____

B. *Clinical Applications*

For the following observations of the oral cavity, a mouth mirror and a piece of gauze are needed.

Review all the structures of the oral cavity so that you will be able to recognize the normal and any deviation from it.

For each structure listed, provide the following information:

- its precise location in the oral cavity
- its clinical appearance (size, shape, color, texture)
- its comparison to the normal

Using the above information as a guide, complete your observations.

1. Vermillion area: Is there cracking? Note any sores. What is the variation in coloring?

2. Philtrum: Note the depth of concavity. How does this affect one's appearance?

3. Maxillary tuberosity: Is this a large projection? What is the condition of the tissue?

4. Retromolar area: Is this mucosa about the same consistency as the buccal mucosa? How large an area is this?

5. Labial frenum: About how many millimeters is this small extension of tissue? Does it extend onto the attached gingiva?

6. Lingual frenum: What is the extent of its length? Is it raised or flat?

7. Buccal frenum: In what position must the jaws be before this can be observed? Which posterior teeth lie adjacent to this?

8. Incisive papilla: Is it raised, flat, inflamed?

9. Palatine rugae: Are they raised or flat? How many pairs are observed?

10. Palatine raphe: How far does this extend along the palate? Is it clearly observed?

11. Fovea palatinus: Are they on the hard or soft palate?

12. Pillars of fauces: Provide another name for the anterior and posterior pillar.

13. Palatine tonsils: Are they present? Describe their position and condition.

14. Uvula: Is it inflamed? What is the length?

15. Tongue: Observe the size, and note whether it is coated. Also locate the papillae: filiform, fungiform, circumvallate, and foliate.

16. Sublingual caruncles: Can you see the duct openings? Describe what the duct openings are like. How high are the caruncles?

17. Buccal mucosa: Is it consistently pink and soft?

18. Stenson's papilla: Which posterior tooth is adjacent to this? Can the opening to the duct be seen?

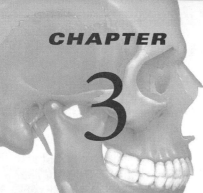

The Tooth and Its Surrounding Structures

KEY TERMS

Crown

Root

Cervix

Anatomic crown

Anatomic root

Clinical crown

Mesial

Distal

Facial

Labial

Buccal

Lingual

Occlusal

Incisal edge

Proximal

Interproximal

Contact area

Apex

Line angle

Point angle

Enamel

Cementum

Dentin

Pulp

Pulp chamber

Pulp horns

Pulp cavity

Apical foramen

Periodontal
ligament

Alveolus

Alveolar process

Lamina dura

Free gingiva

Sulcus

Attached gingiva

Free gingival
junction

Alveolar mucosa

Muco-gingival
junction

Melanin

Divisions of the Tooth
Surfaces of the Tooth
Tissues of the Tooth
The Periodontium

OBJECTIVES

- Identify the divisions of the tooth, surfaces of the tooth, tissues of the tooth, and tissues of the periodontium.
- Describe each tooth tissue and those of the surrounding structures as to location, composition, and function.
- Define the terms noted in boldface.
- Complete the worksheet at the end of the chapter.
- Perform the clinical applications at the end of the chapter.

DIVISIONS OF THE TOOTH

When examining the tooth, note that it is divided into three sections (Figure 3-1).

1. the crown
2. the neck or cervix
3. the root

The **crown** is that portion of the tooth normally visible in the mouth and covered with enamel. The teeth have differently shaped crowns, each adapted to perform a specific function in reducing food for digestion (Figure 3-2).

The **root**, located in the bone and not normally visible, is covered with cementum. Roots stabilize, or support, the teeth when the pressure from mastication is exerted upon them. The crown joins the root at the neck, **cervix**, or cemento-enamel junction (CEJ), a junction between the **anatomic crown** and the **anatomic root**. The anatomic crown is covered with enamel; the anatomic root is covered with cementum. After eruption is complete, only the anatomic crown is seen in the mouth. In later life, as part of the aging process, the gingiva and bone may recede, exposing a portion of the root. All of the tooth that is visible in the mouth, the crown *and* the exposed root together, is referred to as the **clinical crown**. The clinical crown extends from the biting surface of the tooth to the gingival margin.

SURFACES OF THE TOOTH

Every tooth has five surfaces, each surface named according to its position in the arch (Figure 3-3).

Mesial: the surface closest to the midline

Distal: the surface farthest, or most distant, from the midline

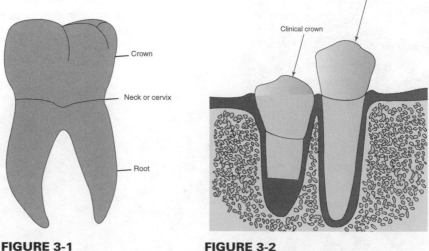

FIGURE 3-1
Divisions of the tooth

FIGURE 3-2
Clinical crown

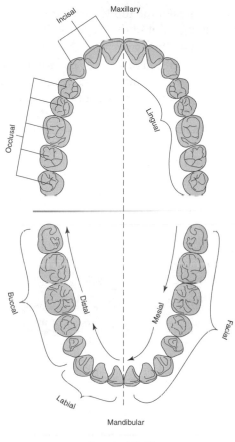

FIGURE 3-3

The surfaces of the teeth identified on the dental arches

Facial: the surfaces closest to the face or outer surfaces of the teeth, including

   Labial: facial surfaces of anterior teeth or surfaces closest to the lip

   Buccal: facial surfaces of posterior teeth or surfaces closest to the cheek

Lingual: surfaces closest to the tongue; all the inner surfaces

Occlusal: chewing surfaces of the posterior teeth

Incisal edge: biting surface of the anterior teeth

Other terms that relate to the surfaces of the teeth are as follows:

Proximal: the surface of the tooth that is next to, or beside, the adjacent tooth. (Mesial and distal surfaces are both proximal surfaces.)

Interproximal: a triangular space between adjacent teeth that is normally filled with the portion of the gingiva called interdental papilla.

Contact area: an area on both the mesial and distal surfaces that touches, or contacts, the adjacent tooth.

Apex: the tip of the root.

Line angle: the area of the tooth where two surfaces meet. For example, the line that joins the buccal and mesial surfaces would be called the mesio-buccal line angle (Figure 3-4).

Point angle: the area of the tooth where three surfaces meet (for example, the joining point of the occlusal, lingual, and mesial surfaces shown in Figure 3-4).

To describe the precise location of an anatomic tooth structure, it is useful to divide the crown and root into thirds as shown in Figure 3-4. Imaginary horizontal lines divide the crown into incisal or occlusal, middle, and cervical thirds and the root into cervical, middle, and apical thirds. Vertical thirds can be used to divide the tooth into mesial, middle, and distal thirds also shown in Figures 3-5, 3-6, 3-7, and 3-8. When explaining details of the tooth, note that a groove can be described as extending to the junction of the occlusal and middle third. This same groove can be located in the distal third of the tooth.

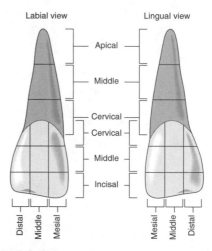

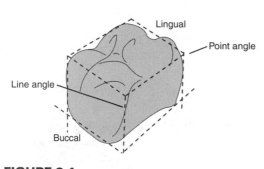

FIGURE 3-4
Point and line angles

FIGURE 3-5
Labial and Lingual views of a maxillary right central incisor, which shows the division of the tooth surfaces in thirds

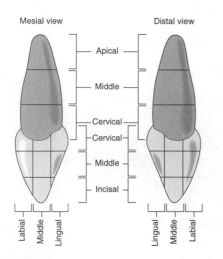

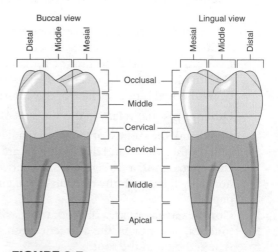

FIGURE 3-6
Mesial and Distal views of a maxillary right central incisor, which shows the division of the tooth surfaces in thirds

FIGURE 3-7
Buccal and Lingual views of a mandibular right molar, which shows the division of the tooth surfaces in thirds

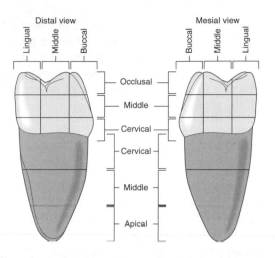

FIGURE 3-8
Mesial and Distal views of a mandibular right molar, which shows the division of the tooth surfaces in thirds

TISSUES OF THE TOOTH

The tissues of the teeth are shown in Figures 3-9 and 3-10 and described below.

Enamel

The crown of the tooth is covered with **enamel,** the hardest tissue in the body. Enamel is made up of 96 percent inorganic (mineral) and 4 percent organic matter and water. It varies in thickness from 2 to 2.5 mm at the biting surface of the tooth to a very thin layer near the cervix. Microscopically,

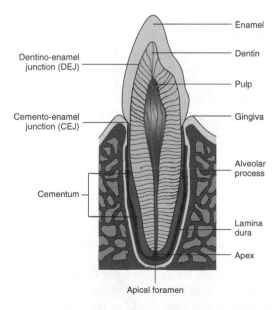

FIGURE 3-9
Tooth and surrounding tissues

the enamel is made up of millions of tiny enamel rods extending from the dentin outwardly, to form the framework of the tooth. Once enamel is complete, it cannot be increased or decreased by the physiologic process. However, it is subject to attrition and dental decay, external processes that occur after the tooth has erupted. Because of its density, enamel is the protective layer of the tooth.

Cementum

Cementum covers the root of the tooth and has the same density as bone. It is 50 percent inorganic and 50 percent organic matter and water. Cementum forms a very thin layer over the root, 0.05 mm or no thicker than a coat of paint on a wall, resulting in its being easily removed during scaling or root planing, or by abrasion when the root is exposed. However, additional cementum can be produced after the eruption of the tooth on areas not exposed in the oral cavity.

Theoretically, the cementum joins the enamel at the cemento-enamel junction. Histologically, however, one of three variations can occur at the cervix:

1. The cementum slightly overlaps the enamel, the most commonly occurring condition.
2. The cementum joins smoothly with enamel.
3. A tiny gap exists between the cementum and the enamel.

Cementum attaches the tooth to the bone by tiny fibers called Sharpey's fibers. These extend from the surrounding periodontal ligament into the cementum.

Dentin

Dentin makes up the major portion of both the crown and the root of the tooth. It is located directly beneath the enamel of the crown and the cementum of the root. Dentin, harder than bone, is 70 percent inorganic and 30 percent organic matter and water. It is made up of an organic matrix, which contains dentinal tubules. The tubules are filled with dentinal fibrils that extend from the pulp to the enamel and carry sensation (temperature, pain) to the pulp.

Pulp

The **pulp** is located at the innermost portion of the tooth and is the only soft tissue of the tooth. It is made up of blood vessels, cellular substances, and nerves.

That pulp structure located in the crown is the **pulp chamber**. It conforms to the shape of the crown, forming small peaks, or **pulp horns**, on the posterior teeth where the crown rises to form cusps (Figure 3-10). The pulp canal is the structure of the pulp located in the root of the tooth. Together, the pulp chamber and the pulp canal make up the **pulp cavity**, a

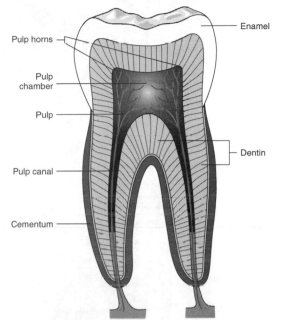

Pulp horns

Pulp chamber

Pulp

Pulp canal

Cementum

Enamel

Dentin

FIGURE 3-10
Tissues of the tooth

space within the center of the tooth. Vessels of the pulp enter and exit the tooth through a small **apical foramen**, or hole, in the apex of the root, where they merge with other similar vessels of the jaw.

The function of the pulp is to assist in the production of dentin, provide sensitivity to the tooth, and act as a defense mechanism by reacting to injury. The pulp also provides nourishment to the tooth.

THE PERIODONTIUM

The periodontium includes those structures that surround and support the teeth (Figure 3-11):

- cementum
- periodontal ligament
- alveolar process
- gingiva

Cementum

Cementum, previously described as a tissue of the tooth, is also considered a supporting structure because it contains fibers extending to the periodontal ligament that hold the tooth in its socket.

Periodontal Ligament

The **periodontal ligament** surrounds the root of the tooth. It is made up of fibers, or ligaments, that support and suspend the tooth in the **alveolus**,

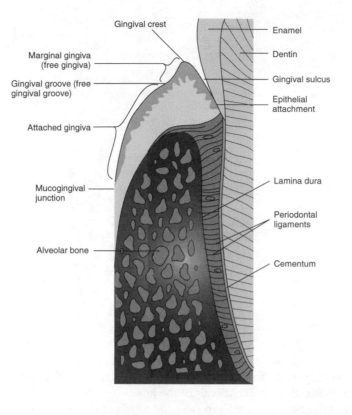

FIGURE 3-11
The periodontium

or socket. Like a tiny trampoline, the fibers, arranged in bundles, act as a shock absorber to keep the tooth from pushing against the bone during the extreme pressure resulting from mastication. Other fibers extend from the periodontal ligament into the cementum on one side and into the alveolar process on the other side to attach the tooth to the bone. These are Sharpey's fibers.

Besides the fibers, the periodontal ligament contains nerves, blood, and lymph vessels. Its function is to produce cementum, stimulate bone resorption, provide sensation upon pressure to the tooth, and provide nutrients through the blood vessels.

Alveolar Process

The **alveolar process** is that portion of the maxilla and mandible that surrounds the roots of the teeth. It is separated from the roots by the periodontal ligament and is made up of bone tissue composed of two layers:

1. cancellous or trabecular bone
2. compact or cortical bone

The inner layer, lightweight and porous, is the trabecular bone. It is surrounded by a denser layer of compact bone structured to endure stress. Compact bone is located adjacent to the periodontal ligament and at the alveolar crest. The layer that surrounds the periodontal ligament forms the

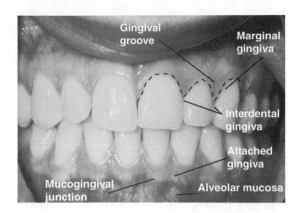

FIGURE 3-12
The periodontium identified on an individual

socket or alveolus of each tooth and is called the **lamina dura**, meaning "hard layer."

Cancellous bone, the innermost layer, is less dense because of the tiny spaces called trabeculae. Without these trabeculae to provide porousness, the bone would be too heavy to move.

The alveolar process supports the tooth and stabilizes the root.

Gingiva

Gingiva, the only portion of the periodontium visible in the oral cavity, is made up of epithelial tissue covered with mucosa (Figures 3-12 and 3-13). It attaches to the underlying bone, surrounds the cervix of the tooth, and fills the interproximal space. It is divided into two sections, free or marginal gingiva and attached gingiva.

Free Gingiva. The gingiva that surrounds the cervix (neck) of the tooth is like a collar and fills the interproximal spaces where it forms the interdental papilla.

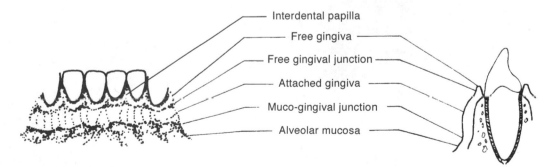

Mandibular incisors
Labial view

Mandibular incisor
Longitudinal section
Proximal view

FIGURE 3-13
Divisions of the gingiva

Free or marginal gingiva is unattached on the inner surface, creating a space or tiny gingival **sulcus** between it and the tooth, as shown in Figure 3-14. The depth of the healthy gingival sulcus is about 1.2 to 1.8 mm before it reaches the epithelial attachment, a layer of cells that merge it with the tooth and the attached gingiva. The gingival sulcus forms a tiny triangle between the free gingiva and the surface of the tooth as its sides and the epithelial attachment as the apex.

Attached gingiva.   This is the portion of the gingiva that can be observed on the external surface. It merges with the free gingiva at the **free gingival junction**, a slight demarcation about 1.2 to 1.8 mm from the gingival crest. The attached gingiva extends apically from the free gingival junction, adhering tightly to the bone beneath it. As compared to other sections of the gingiva, it is pale pink because it is taut to the bone and contains fewer blood vessels.

Attached gingiva extends apically 3.5 to 9.0 mm, where it merges with the **alveolar mucosa** at the **muco-gingival junction**, a scalloped line that follows the contour of the bone.

Gingival description.   Healthy gingiva is pink and stippled (like the skin of an orange) on the attached portion. The color varies with the skin pigmentation so that the darker the skin, the deeper the pink of the gingiva. Occasionally, dark patches of pigmentation, **melanin**, appear on the gingiva of a darker skinned person; these spots of color are normal.

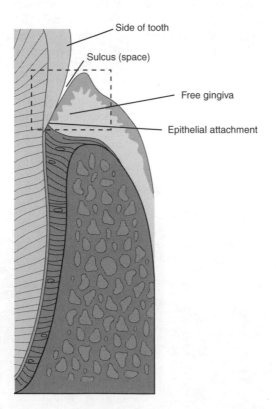

FIGURE 3-14
The gingival sulcus

Normal gingiva is firm and resilient; it follows the contour of the bone and fills the interproximal spaces, forming a sharp, knifelike triangular point at the contact area. Attached gingiva adheres tightly to the bone and is pale, compared to the smooth shiny alveolar mucosa, which contains many blood vessels and thus appears more red in color.

SUMMARY

The integrity of the tooth depends on the good health and stability of all the periodontal tissues. Together, they provide and maintain the longevity of the dentition and protect it from injury.

WORKSHEET

A. Using the following drawing, label the structures listed below.

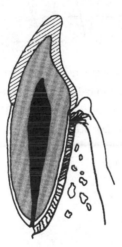

a. Enamel
b. Dentin
c. Pulp canal
d. Cementum
e. Apical foramen

f. Periodontal ligament
g. Cortical bone
h. Trabecular bone
i. Trabecular bone
j. Muco-gingival junction

B. *Clinical Applications*

1. Observe the crowns of the teeth. Record those teeth where the clinical crown is greater than the anatomic crown.

2. Using the illustrations below, draw the height of the free gingiva of the maxillary molars. Draw this on both the buccal and lingual surfaces.

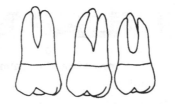

Buccal

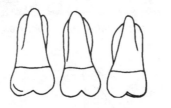

Lingual

3. With an explorer, locate the cervical line (CEJ) of the right molars.

   a. Is the cervical line clinically visible on all teeth?

   b. Is the clinical crown larger or smaller than the anatomic crown?

4. Observe the gingiva. Locate and describe the following sections as they appear in the oral cavity:

   a. Marginal (free) gingiva

   b. Interdental papilla

   c. Attached gingiva

   d. Muco-gingival line

   e. Alveolar mucosa

5. Use a periodontal probe to feel the depth and continuity of the gingival sulcus around teeth #6–8 and #30.

   a. What is the approximate depth of a normal sulcus? _____

   b. What is the sulcus depth of the teeth just explored?

   #6 _____   #7 _____   #8 _____   #30 _____

6. Observe the occlusal surfaces and note that they are not smooth. They have pits and grooves. Follow these grooves, gently, with an explorer. If the explorer sticks, record the tooth and surface below.

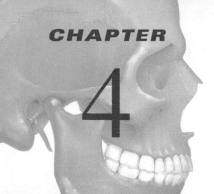

Numbering Systems

The Universal Numbering System
Palmer's Notation
Federation Dentaire Internationale (FDI)/
   International Standards Organization/(ISO)

OBJECTIVES

- Identify three different numbering systems.
- Describe each numbering system as to its designation of dentition, arch, quadrant, and tooth.
- Complete the worksheet at the end of the chapter.
- Perform the clinical applications at the end of the chapter.

THE UNIVERSAL NUMBERING SYSTEM

Permanent Teeth

In the United States, the Universal Numbering System is the most widely accepted method used to record teeth. It is uncomplicated and efficient. Each tooth is numbered from 1 to 32 in consecutive order beginning with the patient's maxillary right third molar as tooth #1 and continuing to the maxillary left third molar as tooth #16 (Figure 4-1). The numbers continue on the mandibular left side with the mandibular left third molar, tooth #17, and follow consecutively to the mandibular right third molar, tooth #32.

Primary Teeth

The primary teeth are numbered consecutively in the same manner as the permanent teeth from the maxillary right second molar to the maxillary left second molar using the letter "A" for the primary maxillary right second molar and "J" for the primary maxillary left second molar (Figure 4-2).

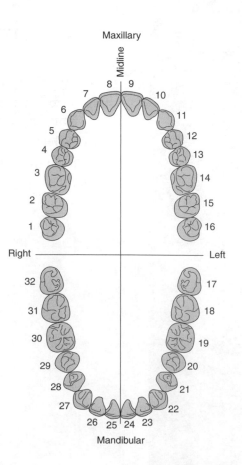

FIGURE 4-1

Universal Numbering System—permanent dentition

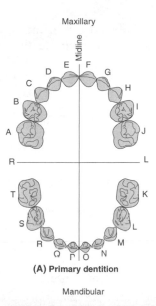

Maxillary

(A) Primary dentition

Mandibular

FIGURE 4-2
Universal Numbering
System—primary dentition

PALMER'S NOTATION

Palmer's Notation designates each tooth according to its location in a quadrant. A horizontal line separates the maxilla from the mandible and a vertical midline separates the patient's right and left sides of the mouth, as shown in Figure 4-3.

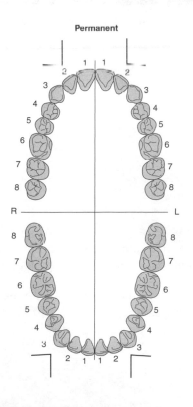

Permanent

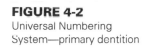

Primary

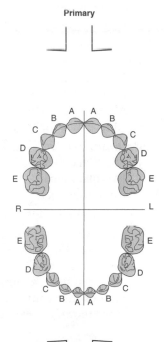

FIGURE 4-3
Palmer's Notation—
permanent and primary
dentitions

Permanent teeth are numbered 1–8 in each quadrant, beginning at the central incisor to the third molar. Primary teeth are designated with the letters A–E.

When identifying an individual tooth, use a right angle to specify the quadrant and arch, as follows:

maxillary right	maxillary left
mandibular right	mandibular left

The tooth number is written within the angle:

Permanent maxillary right central incisor   1|

Permanent mandibular left first premolar |4

Primary maxillary left second molar |E

Primary mandibular right canine   C|

FEDERATION DENTAIRE INTERNATIONALE (FDI)/INTERNATIONAL STANDARDS ORGANIZATION (ISO)

The FDI/ISO numbering system was introduced to provide a standard international system of coding teeth (Figure 4-4). Each quadrant is assigned a number:

Permanent Teeth
Maxillary right	1
Maxillary left	2
Mandibular left	3
Mandibular right	4

Primary Teeth
Maxillary right	5
Maxillary left	6
Mandibular left	7
Mandibular right	8

The teeth within each quadrant are then numbered 1–8, from the central incisor to the third molar, as with Palmer's Notation. The primary teeth are numbered 1–5.

To use this system, identify each tooth with a two-digit figure: the first digit designates the dentition, arch, and quadrant; the second digit codes the individual tooth. For example:

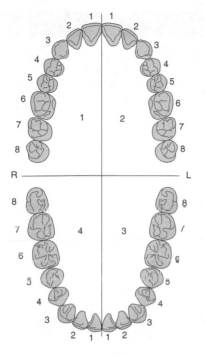

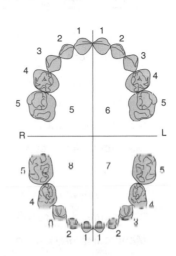

FIGURE 4-4
Federation Dentaire
Internationale (FDI)/
International Standards
Organization (ISO)

Permanent Maxillary right	→ 1	3 ←	canine	13
Permanent Mandibular left	→ 3	1 ←	central incisor	31
Primary Maxillary left	→ 6	4 ←	first molar	64
Primary Mandibular right	→ 8	2 ←	lateral incisor	82

SUMMARY

The three numbering systems described—Palmer's Notation, the Universal Numbering System, and the Federation Dentaire Internationale (FDI)/International Standards Organization (ISO) are the most commonly used standards for identifying and charting teeth. Numbering systems provide a basis for coding the conditions of the teeth in a manner that is efficient and convenient for dental personnel.

WORKSHEET

A. Identify the appropriate code for each tooth listed.

	Universal Number	Palmer's Notation	FDI/ISO
Permanent Teeth			
Maxillary right second molar			
Maxillary left canine			
Maxillary left central incisor			
Mandibular left first premolar			
Mandibular right canine			
Maxillary right lateral incisor			
Mandibular right second molar			
Mandibular left first molar			
Deciduous Teeth			
Mandibular right canine			
Maxillary left second molar			
Mandibular left central incisor			
Maxillary right lateral incisor			
Mandibular left first molar			

B. Clinical Applications

1. Observe the teeth in each quadrant and record those that are missing by using the following numbering systems.

   a. Universal Numbering System

   b. Palmer's Notation

   c. FDI/ISO

2. Observe the maxillary first molar. Record its antagonist(s) by using the Universal Numbering System.

3. Record the left premolars using Palmer's Notation. Using the same recording method, note the deciduous teeth that precede the premolars.

4. Using the Universal Numbering System, record the third tooth from the midline and the fourth tooth from the midline, both maxillary and mandibular. Are these the same teeth in the permanent and deciduous dentition?

5. Record the first permanent tooth to erupt using the Universal Number.

6. Which tooth replaces R?

7. Compare the crowns of #9 and #10.

INTRODUCTORY INFORMATION

After you have finished this section, you will be able to identify the location in the dental arch of each anterior tooth (Figure II-1), as well as its universal number, expected eruption date, usual crown and root completion dates, function, lengths of crown and root, antagonists, location of contact areas, number of lobes, and pulp canals. You will be able to state at what age there is evidence of calcification during the formation of each tooth.

You will be able to describe the location and/or contour of the incisal edge or cusp slopes, the mesial and distal outlines, contact areas, surface characteristics, the developmental depressions, root shape, cervical lines, and lingual structures. Use Appendix D to compare the depth of the cervical lines of the teeth and to identify the location of the root depressions.

You will also be able to define terms such as **anomaly**, **cingulum**, **developmental depression**, **fossa**, **groove**, **lobe**, **pit**, and **root depression**.

Certain characteristics and structures are common to all anterior teeth. To assist in understanding the tooth morphology, and to avoid repetition throughout the chapters, the following related information provides a general background applicable to all anterior teeth.

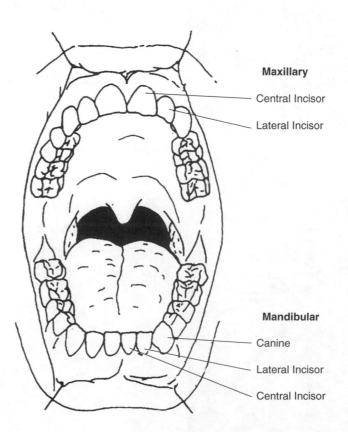

Maxillary

Central Incisor

Lateral Incisor

Mandibular

Canine

Lateral Incisor

Central Incisor

FIGURE II-1

Permanent anterior teeth

Related Information

Lobe. A center of development and calcification from which a tooth is formed. All anterior teeth develop from four lobes that eventually coalesce to shape the crown. Three lobes form a labial surface of the crown and the fourth lobe shapes a cingulum on the lingual surface. Lines of demarcation from lobe coalescence are evident as linear depressions on the labial surface.

Mamelons. Structures that make up a scalloped border along the incisal edge of the incisors and are present at the eruption of the teeth. Mamelons are remnants of lobe formation that are worn away by attrition shortly after eruption (Figure II-2).

Cervical Line. (Also known as the cemento-enamel junction, or CEJ). A demarcation separating the anatomic crown and root. When the tooth is viewed from the labial or lingual surface, the cervical line appears as a semicircle curving toward the root. From the proximal surface, the cervical line curves incisally. Its depth varies from 1 to 3 mm; this is significant when the teeth are being scaled. For further information on this subject, see Chapter 16.

Col Area. A depression of the interdental papilla on the proximal surfaces of the teeth. The papillae form a "U" shape cervical to the contact area of each tooth.

Root Apex. The tip of the root. In most instances, the root tip of an anterior tooth has a distal inclination. The exception is the mandibular canine, which frequently has a mesially inclined root tip.

Apical Foramen. A tiny opening in the apex of the root of the tooth through which blood vessels and nerves exit and enter.

Pulp Canal. A structure containing the pulp that is located in the root of the tooth. All anterior teeth have one root and one pulp canal.

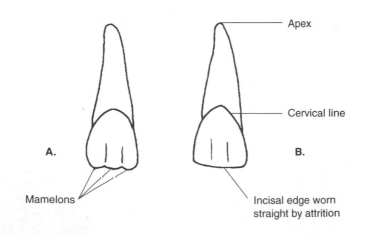

A.

B.

Apex

Cervical line

Mamelons

Incisal edge worn straight by attrition

FIGURE II-2

Maxillary right central incisor—labial surface

Antagonist.   A tooth that contacts another tooth in the opposite arch. Mandibular teeth contact maxillary teeth; they are the antagonists of each other. All anterior teeth have two antagonists *except* the mandibular central incisors, which have only one (Figure II-3).

Succedaneous Tooth.   A permanent tooth that replaces, or succeeds, a primary tooth in the same position. Each permanent anterior tooth succeeds a primary anterior tooth; for example, the permanent maxillary central incisor succeeds the primary maxillary central incisor (Figure II-4). The permanent incisor is the succedaneous tooth.

Structures Common to All Anterior Teeth

Fossa.   A shallow rounded depression.

Ridge.   A linear elevation. Ridges are named by their location—for example, the mesial marginal ridge or lingual ridge.

Cingulum.   A convex, or rounded, elevation or tubercle on the cervical third of the lingual surface. This is a remnant of the fourth, or lingual, lobe.

Root Depression or Furrow.   A shallow, linear concavity located on either the crown or root.

Pit.   A pinpoint depression.

FIGURE II-3
All anterior teeth have two antagonists except the mandibular central incisor

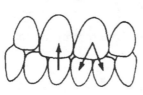

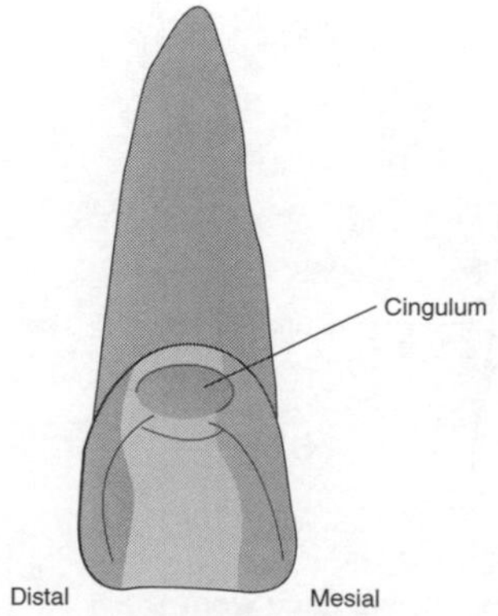

FIGURE II-4
Maxillary central incisor—lingual surface

Cingulum

Distal   Mesial

Maxillary Incisors

General Information
Maxillary Central Incisor
Maxillary Lateral Incisor

OBJECTIVES

- Identify the maxillary incisors and provide vital information: that is, universal number, function, antagonist, and so forth.
- Describe the location and contour of each maxillary incisor.
- Define the new terms in the chapter.
- Complete the worksheet at the end of the chapter.

GENERAL INFORMATION

There are four maxillary incisors: two central and two lateral incisors. Each quadrant has only one central incisor and one lateral incisor. Both the central and lateral incisors are similar in shape; however, the lateral incisor is smaller and slightly more convex. See Figure 5-1 for a comparison of the size of the maxillary central incisor.

At eruption, mamelons are more prominent on the central incisor, but they are normally worn away by attrition after a short period of use. Incisors are wedge-shaped from the proximal view (see Figure 5-7) with a straight, sharp cutting, or incisal, edge that makes them adaptable for incising food.

This text describes the "ideal" morphology of each tooth. Actual teeth will show variations, which are normal. Occasionally there is an extreme deviation from the norm. This is called an **anomaly**.

A frequent deviation of the maxillary central incisor is a variation in root length, the most common of which is a short or blunted root.

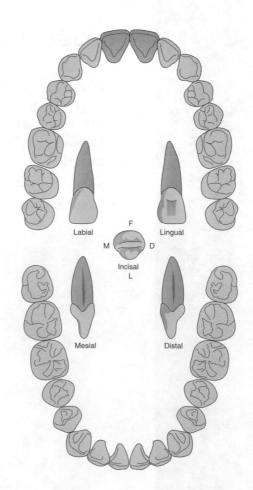

FIGURE 5-1
Maxillary central incisors

The maxillary lateral incisor is the tooth, other than third molars, that most commonly forms as an anomaly. Its most frequent variation of crown shape is the "peg-shaped" lateral.

MAXILLARY CENTRAL INCISOR

Characteristics

Location in the Arch . . . . One on either side of midline
Universal Number . . . . R-#8   L-#9
Eruption Date . . . . 7–8 years
First Evidence of Calcification . . . . . 3–4 months
Crown Completion . . . . 4–5 years
Root Completion . . . . 10 years
Function . . . . Biting, incising
Length of Crown . . . . 10.5 mm
Length of Root . . . . 13 mm
Antagonists . . . . Mandibular central and lateral
                                             incisors

Location of Contact Area

Mesial . . . . Mesio-incisal angle
Distal . . . . Slightly cervical to
                                             disto-incisal angle

Identifying Features

- widest anterior tooth mesio-distally
- straight mesial side with sharp mesio-incisal angle and convex distal side
- straight incisal edge
- wedge shape of tooth from proximal view

(Refer to Figure 5-1)

Tooth Description of the Maxillary Central Incisor

Labial Surface.   After the **mamelons** are worn away the incisal edge is straight, slightly inclining toward the distal side of the tooth. The mesio-incisal angle is sharp, contacting the mesial of the adjacent central incisor at the incisal edge. Tapering gradually, the mesial side continues straight until it merges with the cervical line. The disto-incisal angle, slightly rounded, forms the distal contact area in the incisal third. The distal side of the tooth is slightly convex, tapering until it joins the cervical line, a semicircle. Two slight vertical **developmental depressions**, the result of lobe formation, are present on the labial surface; otherwise it is smooth. A cone-shaped root tapers gradually to a blunt apex (Figure 5-2).

Lingual Surface.   The outline of the lingual surface is the reverse of the labial view. A well-defined **lingual fossa** is outlined by mesial and distal

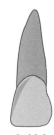

Labial

FIGURE 5-2
Maxillary central incisor—labial surface

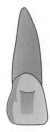

FIGURE 5-3

Maxillary central incisor—lingual surface

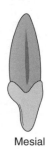

FIGURE 5-4

Maxillary central incisor—mesial and distal surfaces

marginal ridges and the **cingulum** (Figure 5-3). Frequently, shallow grooves are found in the fossa. A pronounced cingulum dominates the cervical third of the crown.

Proximal Surfaces.   Seen from this view is a typical wedge shape that renders the tooth adaptable for biting and incising food. Note that the **cervical line** curves incisally for about one-third the length of the crown (Figure 5-4).

The root is broad and smooth (with no depressions or furrows) and tapers, in the apical third, to a blunt apex. The tip of the root and the incisal edge are on the midline, providing balance for the tooth when functioning.

CLINICAL CONSIDERATIONS
Root length: 13 mm
Root depressions/furrows: None
CEJ: Curves incisally 2.5–3.5 mm
Cervical area: Smooth

Summary of the Maxillary Central Incisor

Labial Surface.   The characteristics of this surface are as follows:

- A straight incisal edge, inclining toward distal.
- A straight mesial side.
- A sharp mesio-incisal angle.
- A mesial contact area (X) located at the mesio-incisal angle.
- A slightly convex distal side.
- A rounded disto-incisal angle.
- A distal contact area (X) located in the incisal third.
- Developmental depressions on the crown.
- A cone-shaped root with a blunt apex.

Lingual Surface.   The characteristics of this surface are as follows:

- An outline that is the reverse of the labial.
- A concave lingual fossa.
- Mesial and distal marginal ridges that outline the fossa.
- A convex cingulum that makes up the cervical third of the crown.

Proximal Surfaces.   The characteristics of these surfaces are as follows:

- A cervical line that curves one-third of the tooth toward the incisal (3 mm on mesial, 2 mm on the distal).
- The tip of the incisal edge and the root located on the midline.
- A root that is broad and tapers in the apical third.
- No furrows or depressions on the root.

MAXILLARY LATERAL INCISOR

Characteristics

Location in the Arch . . . . Distal to central incisor; second
tooth from midline
Universal Number . . . . R-#7   L-#10
Eruption Date . . . . 8–9 years
First Evidence of Calcification . . . . . 1 year
Crown Completion . . . . 4–5 years
Root Completion . . . . 11 years
Function . . . . Biting, incising
Length of Crown . . . . 9 mm
Length of Root . . . . 13 mm
Antagonists . . . . Mandibular lateral incisor and
canine

Location of Contact Area

Mesial . . . . Junction of middle and
incisal third
Distal . . . . Middle third

Identifying Features

- resembles maxillary central incisor but is smaller, with more
convex mesial and distal sides and incisal angles
- developmental variations are frequent

(Refer to Figure 5-1)

Tooth Description of the Maxillary Lateral Incisor

Labial Surface.   The lateral incisor has the same shape as the central
incisor but is smaller and slightly more convex (Figure 5-6). The incisal
edge inclines toward the distal. Both the mesial and distal incisal angles are
rounded, and both the mesial and distal sides of the tooth are convex. As
compared to the mesial, the distal outline is more convex and the angle
more rounded. Although developmental depressions may be present, the
labial surface is usually smooth. Both mesial and distal contact areas are
located more cervically than on the central incisor. A cone-shaped root
tapers, gradually, toward the apex.

Lingual Surface.   The lingual outline is the reverse of the labial (Figure 5-7). However, the cingulum is very pronounced, and a developmental
pit is often located in the fossa directly beneath it. The lingual fossa is more
likely to have developmental grooves than the maxillary central incisor. All
other structures are the same as those of the central incisor.

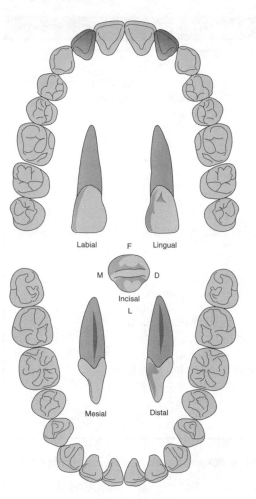

FIGURE 5-5
Maxillary lateral incisors

Maxillary lateral incisors

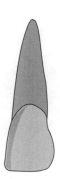

Labial

FIGURE 5-6
Maxillary lateral incisor—
labial surface

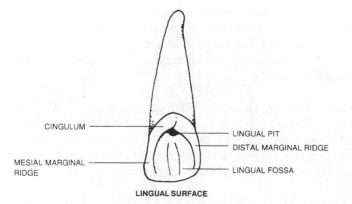

FIGURE 5-7
Maxillary lateral incisor—lingual surface

Proximal Surfaces. The structures and shape, from this view, are the same as the maxillary central incisor. However, there is often a furrow, or long, shallow depression, present on the root (Figure 5-8).

CLINICAL CONSIDERATIONS
Root length: 13 mm
Root depressions/furrows: Mesial and distal vertical depressions usually present
CEJ: Curves incisally 2–3 mm
Cervical area: May have shallow concavity

Summary of the Maxillary Lateral Incisor

Labial Surface. The characteristics of this surface are:

- A straight incisal edge that inclines toward the distal.
- Rounded mesial and distal incisal angles.
- Convex mesial and distal sides.
- Mesial and distal contact areas that are more cervical than the central incisor.
- A smooth labial surface.
- A tapered root.

Lingual Surface. The characteristics of this surface are:

- A prominent cingulum.
- A developmental pit usually in the fossa below the cingulum.

Proximal Surface. The characteristics of this surface are:

- A wedged-shaped outline that is the same as the maxillary central incisor.
- A cervical line that curves one-third of the tooth toward the incisal.
- A broad root with furrows on both the mesial and distal surfaces.

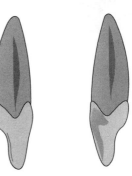

Mesial   Distal

FIGURE 5-8
Maxillary lateral incisor—mesial and distal surfaces

SUMMARY

Incisors are wedge-shaped teeth with sharp, straight incisal edges used to cut or incise food. Both the maxillary central and lateral incisors have similar shapes, although the lateral incisor is smaller and slightly more convex.

WORKSHEET

A. *Complete the following chart with the information requested.*

	Central Incisor	Lateral Incisor
Universal Number		
Palmer's Notation		
Eruption Date		
Antagonists		
Anomalies		
Location of Contact Area		
Mesial		
Distal		
Succedaneous		
Number of Lobes		
*Labial Depressions**		
*Lingual**		
Ridges		
Cingulum		
Fossa		
Root Shape and Depressions		
Labial		
Proximal		

*Indicate location, size, and/or shape

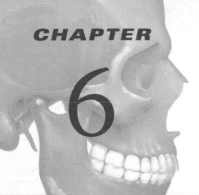

Mandibular Incisors

General Information
Mandibular Central Incisor
Mandibular Lateral Incisor

OBJECTIVES

- Identify the mandibular incisors and provide vital information: that is, universal number, function, antagonist, and so forth.
- Describe the location and contour of each mandibular incisor.
- Define the new terms in the chapter.
- Complete the worksheet at the end of the chapter.

GENERAL INFORMATION

There are four mandibular incisors: two central incisors and two lateral incisors. Each quadrant has one central and one lateral incisor.

The central and lateral incisors appear quite similar although the lateral incisor is larger. The opposite situation exists in the maxilla, where the central is larger than the lateral incisor.

As the smallest tooth in the dentition, the mandibular central incisor has only one **antagonist** (Figure 6-1). This tooth and the maxillary third molar are the only teeth that have one antagonist; all others have two.

Shortly after eruption, mamelons are usually worn away by attrition and the incisal edges of all incisors are straight. Viewed from the proximal surface, the mandibular incisors have the same wedge shape as the maxillary incisors, and so are suited, also, for incising food.

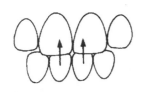

FIGURE 6-1

The mandibular central incisor has only one antagonist

MANDIBULAR CENTRAL INCISOR

Characteristics

Location in the Arch	One, on either side of the mid-line
Universal Number.	R-#25 L-#24
Eruption Date.	6–7 years
First Evidence of Calcification	3–4 months
Crown Completion	4–5 years
Root Completion	9 years
Function	Incising, biting
Length of Crown	9 mm
Length of Root	12.5 mm
Antagonist	Maxillary central incisor

Location of Contact Area

Mesial	Mesial incisal angle
Distal	Distal incisal angle

Identifying Features

- smallest tooth in the oral cavity
- bilaterally symmetric from labial or lingual view
- smooth tooth; no developmental grooves or depression in crown
- only one antagonist

Tooth Description of the Mandibular Central Incisor

Labial Surface.   The incisal edge is straight, joining the mesial and distal sides at sharp incisal angles. These angles are the contact areas. Both mesial and distal sides are straight, tapering evenly to the cervix where the cervical line forms an arc.

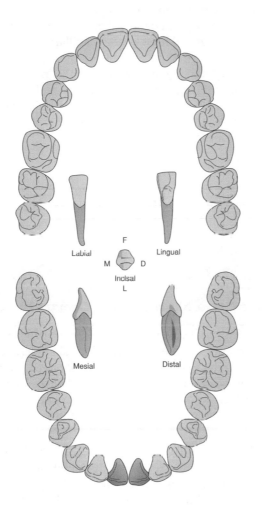

Labial   Lingual

F

M   D

Incisal

L

Mesial   Distal

FIGURE 6-2
Mandibular central incisors

The tooth is **bilaterally symmetric**—the same on both sides—so it is difficult to differentiate the mesial from the distal side. The root is straight, tapering gradually to the apex (Figure 6-2).

Lingual Surface. The outline from the lingual is the reverse of the labial view. This surface is very smooth; there are no pits or grooves and the **fossa** and cingulum merge with a gentle curve. Marginal ridges are not evident, as is the case with maxillary incisors. The cingulum covers the cervical third of the crown; the smooth, shallow fossa occupies the remaining two-thirds (Figure 6-3).

Proximal Surfaces. The width, from labial to lingual, is broad to compensate for the narrow mesial to distal measurements seen from the labial view. The width is necessary to provide stability, in the bone, for such a small tooth. The root remains broad for two-thirds its length, tapering only at the apical third. Both the mesial and distal root surfaces have a deep depression extending most of the root length (Figure 6-2).

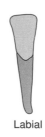

Labial

FIGURE 6-3
Mandibular central incisor—labial surface

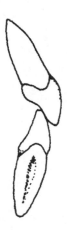

FIGURE 6-4
Mandibular right incisors—
lingual surface

The incisal edge of the mandibular incisor is positioned lingual to the midline. When the teeth occlude, the labial surface of the mandibular incisors conforms to the lingual fossa of the maxillary incisors (Figure 6-4).

Incisal View. Observing this tooth from the incisal aspect assists in differentiating it from the mandibular lateral incisor. The central incisor has a straight incisal edge that is bilaterally symmetric (Figure 6-5). Usually, it is difficult to distinguish the mesial side from the distal side of the crown because of their similarity in structure.

CLINICAL CONSIDERATIONS
Root length: 12.5 mm
Root depressions/furrows: Deep vertical depressions on both mesial and distal surfaces
CEJ: Curves incisally 2–3 mm
Cervical area: May have shallow concavity on both mesial and distal surfaces

Summary of the Mandibular Central Incisor

Labial Surface. The characteristics of this surface are:
- A straight incisal edge with sharp incisal angles.
- Mesial and distal sides that taper evenly to the cervix.
- Mesial and distal contact areas located at the incisal angle.
- A smooth crown surface with no depressions.
- A straight root, tapering at the apical third.

Lingual Surface. The characteristics of this surface are:
- An outline that is the reverse of the labial view.
- A smooth fossa; a smooth cingulum.
- A convex cingulum that is one-third of the crown.

Proximal Surfaces. The characteristics of these surfaces are:
- The tip of the incisal edge sitting lingual to the midline.
- A cervical line that curves toward the incisal edge.
- A broad root, tapering at the apical third.
- A root furrow or depression on the mesial and distal surfaces.

Incisal View. The characteristics of this surface are:
- A straight incisal ridge.
- A bilaterally symmetric form.

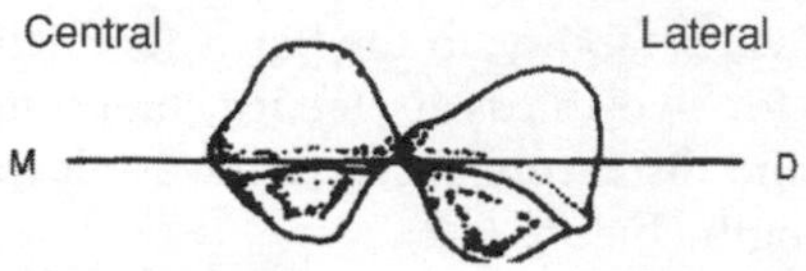

Central   Lateral

M ———   ——— D

FIGURE 6-5
Mandibular incisors—
incisal view

MANDIBULAR LATERAL INCISOR

Characteristics

Location in the Arch	Distal to central incisor; second tooth from midline
Universal Number	R-#26 L-#23
Eruption Date	7–8 years
First Evidence of Calcification	3–4 months
Crown Completion	4–5 years
Root Completion	10 years
Function	Biting, incising
Length of Crown	9.5 mm
Length of Root	14 mm
Antagonists	Maxillary central and lateral incisors

Location of Contact Area

Mesial	Mesial incisal angle
Distal	Cervical to the incisal angle

Identifying Features

- slightly larger than the central incisor
- slightly more convex than the central incisor
- incisal ridge curves to the distal
- crown distally displaced

Tooth Description of the Mandibular Lateral Incisor

Labial Surface.   The lateral incisor looks like the central incisor in overall appearance but is slightly larger and not bilaterally symmetric. Whereas the central incisor has a level incisal edge, the incisal edge of the lateral declines toward the distal and forms a rounded incisal angle with the distal side. The distal side is slightly convex. The mesial incisal angle is sharp; the mesial side can be straight or slightly convex as it tapers toward the cervical line. Both the mesial and distal contact areas are at the incisal angle. The cervical line forms a narrow arch. The root is straight, tapering at the apical third (Figure 6-6).

Lingual and Proximal Surfaces.   Except for size and length, the mandibular lateral incisor is similar to the central incisor and has the same characteristics. However, the cingulum is distally displaced as it starts to curve toward the canine (Figures 6-6 and 6-7).

Incisal View.   The incisal edge of the lateral incisor curves toward the distal, following the contour of the mandibular arch, whereas the incisal edge of the central incisor is straight. The curvature on the lateral incisor creates a distally displaced cingulum as compared to the centrally situated cingulum of the central incisor. This structure assists in distinguishing the two teeth from each other (Figure 6-5).

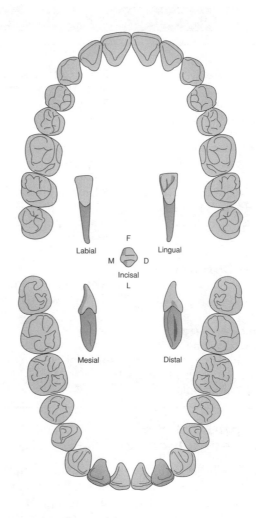

FIGURE 6-6
Mandibular lateral incisors

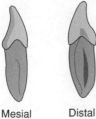

FIGURE 6-7
Mandibular lateral incisor—
mesial and distal surface

CLINICAL CONSIDERATIONS
Root length: 14 mm
Root depressions/furrows: Both mesial and distal with deeper distal depression
CEJ: Curves incisally 2–3 mm
Cervical area: May have shallow concavity

Summary of the Mandibular Lateral Incisor

Labial Surface.   The characteristics of this surface are:

- An incisal edge that declines toward the distal.
- A mesial surface that tapers gradually toward the cervix.
- A distal side that is slightly convex, tapering toward the cervix.
- A sharp mesial incisal angle; a rounded distal incisal angle.
- Mesial and distal contact areas at the junction of the incisal edge and the mesial or distal side.

- A smooth surface.
- A straight root that tapers evenly.

Lingual Surface.   The characteristics of this surface are:
- An outline that is the reverse of the labial side.
- Cingulum, fossa, and ridges that appear the same as those on the central incisor.

Proximal Surfaces.   The characteristics of these surfaces are:
- Root depressions on the mesial and distal surfaces; the distal depression is deeper.
- All other characteristics that are the same as those pertaining to the central incisor.

Incisal View.   The characteristics of this view are:
- An incisal edge that curves toward the distal and inward toward the lingual.
- A cingulum that is distally displaced.

SUMMARY

Mandibular incisors assist the maxillary incisors in biting and cutting food. From the labial view, both mandibular incisors are small, narrow teeth with a straight incisal edge and tapering mesial and distal sides. The mandibular central incisor is the smallest tooth in the dentition.

WORKSHEET

A. Complete the following chart with the information requested.

	Central Incisor	Lateral Incisor
Universal Number		
Palmer's Notation		
Eruption Date		
Antagonists		
Anomalies		
Location of Contact Area		
Mesial		
Distal		
Succedaneous		
Number of Lobes		
*Labial Depressions**		
*Lingual**		
Ridges		
Cingulum		
Fossa		
Root Shape and Depressions		
Labial		
Proximal		

*Indicate location, size, and/or shape

Canines

General Information

Maxillary Canine

Mandibular Canine

OBJECTIVES

- Identify the canines and provide vital information: that is, universal number, function, antagonist, and so forth.
- Describe the location and contour of each canine.
- Define the new terms in the chapter.
- Complete the worksheet at the end of the chapter.
- Complete the clinical applications at the end of the chapter.

GENERAL INFORMATION

There are two canines in each arch: one in each quadrant. Maxillary and mandibular canines are similar, with variations as noted in the descriptions. Both maxillary and mandibular canines have a sharp, pointed cusp, thus attaining their alternate name of "**cuspids**." They are long, strong, stable teeth. Note their size and length (Figure 7-1) as compared to the adjacent teeth. Canines usually have one root. However, with variation, the mandibular canine may have two roots, and thus two pulp canals.

Because they are located at the corner of each arch, canines are referred to as the "**cornerstone**" teeth. Their position is important to **aesthetics** because they provide shape to the face. If dentures are needed and the size or position of the canine is varied, the entire facial appearance can change. Fortunately, canines are self-cleansing, because of their convexity and location at the corners of the arch, so that food easily rolls off them. Thus, they are usually the last teeth to be lost by dental decay. The shape of this tooth, particularly the sharp cusp, makes it adaptable for holding and tearing food.

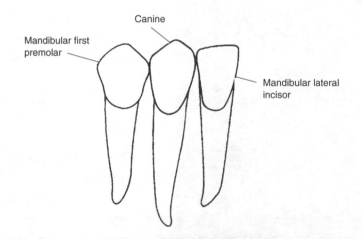

FIGURE 7-1

Mandibular canine with proximal teeth

MAXILLARY CANINE

Characteristics

Location in the Arch	Distal to lateral incisor; third tooth from midline
Universal Number	R-#6 L-#11
Eruption Date	11–12 years
First Evidence of Calcification	4–5 months
Crown Completion	6–7 years
Root Completion	13–15 years
Function	Tearing, holding
Length of Crown	10 mm
Length of Root	17 mm
Antagonist	Mandibular canine and first premolar

(continues)

MAXILLARY CANINE (continued)

Location of Contact Area

Mesial . . . . Junction of incisal and middle third

Distal . . . . Middle third

Identifying Features

- longest maxillary tooth
- stable, sturdy tooth
- cornerstone of the arch
- sharp, pointed cusp
- bulky cingulum and defined lingual ridges

(Refer to Figure 7-2)

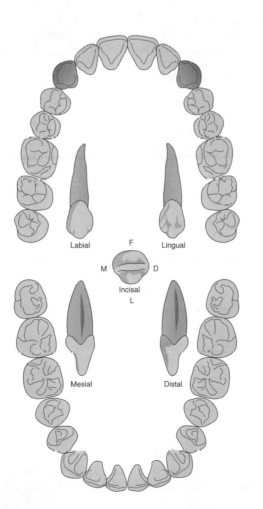

FIGURE 7-2
Maxillary canines

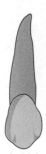

Labial

FIGURE 7-3
Maxillary canine—labial
surface

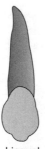

Lingual

FIGURE 7-4
Maxillary canine—lingual
surface

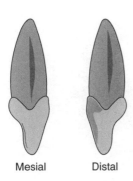

Mesial   **Distal**

FIGURE 7-5
Maxillary canine—mesial and
distal surfaces

Tooth Description of the Maxillary Canine

Labial Surface.   The area extending from the tip of the cusp to both the mesial and distal contact areas is called a **cusp slope**. Both contact areas are located near the junction of the incisal and middle third of the tooth. The mesial cusp slope is shorter than the distal cusp slope. It joins the mesial surface at the junction of the incisal and middle third; the mesial side is convex. Because of the longer cusp slope, the distal contact area is more cervical than the mesial and is located in the middle third of the crown. The distal side of the tooth is slightly concave before merging with the cervical line.

A well-developed middle lobe, called the **labial ridge**, is centrally located and extends from the cervix to the tip of the cusp. Shallow depressions extend, vertically, along both sides of the ridge. The root is cone-shaped and usually smooth (Figure 7-3).

Lingual Surface.   The outline is the reverse of the labial view, but narrower. Forming the lingual surface are two fossae and a well-pronounced cingulum (Figure 7-4). The cingulum is situated in the cervical third of the crown. A **lingual ridge** divides the **lingual fossa** into two segments—a mesial lingual fossa and a distal lingual fossa—and extends from the base of the cingulum to the cusp tip. Raised mesial and distal marginal ridges outline the lateral border of the fossae.

Proximal Surfaces.   Both the length and width of the maxillary canine, as seen from the proximal surfaces, are greater than other anterior teeth (Figure 7-5). This width is needed to give the tooth stability. The root is broad for two-thirds its length, tapering only at the apical third. Deep depressions on the mesial and distal root surfaces give the tooth greater stability in the bone, needed during mastication.

CLINICAL CONSIDERATIONS
Root length: 17 mm
Root depressions/furrows: Deep depressions on both mesial and distal surfaces
CEJ: Curves incisally 1.5–2.5 mm on mesial and distal surfaces
Cervical area: Concave on both mesial and distal surfaces

Summary of the Maxillary Canine

Labial Surface.   The characteristics of this surface are:

- A mesial cusp slope that is shorter than the distal cusp slope.
- A mesial contact area that is at the junction of the incisal and the middle third.
- A distal contact area that is in the middle third of the tooth.
- A slightly convex mesial side.
- Slightly concave from cervix to contact area on distal side.
- A well-developed middle lobe, called the labial ridge.

- Depressions that are on either side of the labial ridge.
- A cusp tip that is centered over the root.
- A cone-shaped, smooth root.

Lingual Surface.   The characteristics of this surface are:

- An outline that is the reverse of the labial view.
- A crown and root that converge so that both mesial and distal surfaces can be seen.
- A fossa that is divided, by a lingual ridge, into mesio-lingual and disto-lingual fossae.
- A pronounced cingulum and marginal ridges.

Proximal Surfaces.   The characteristics of these surfaces are:

- A broad crown and root.
- A cervical line that curves toward the incisal.
- A deep depression in the root surface.

MANDIBULAR CANINE

Characteristics

Location in the Arch	Distal to lateral incisor; third tooth from midline
Universal Number.	R-#27 L-#22
Eruption Date.	9–10 years
First Evidence of Calcification	4–5 months
Crown Completion	6–7 years
Root Completion	12–14 years
Function	Tearing, holding
Length of Crown	11 mm
Length of Root.	16 mm
Antagonists	Maxillary lateral incisor and canine

Location of Contact Area

Mesial	Incisal third
Distal	Junction of incisal and middle third

Identifying Features

- longest mandibular tooth
- well-developed middle lobe called labial ridge
- slightly narrower and smoother than maxillary canine

(Refer to Figure 7-6)

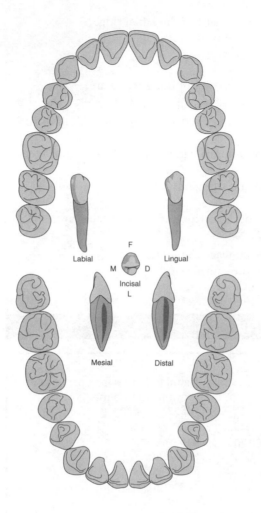

FIGURE 7-6
Mandibular canines

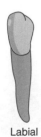

Labial

FIGURE 7-7
Mandibular canine—labial
surface

Tooth Description of the Mandibular Canine

Labial Surface. The crown of the mandibular canine looks similar to that of the maxillary canine but is narrower by 0.5 mm. It appears even narrower than this, as compared to the maxillary canine, because both the mesial and distal contact areas are located more incisally.

The mesial cusp slope is shorter than the distal; the mesial side of the tooth is straight, whereas the distal side is more convex (Figure 7-7). The labial ridge is not as prominent as on the maxillary canine, and there are depressions on either side of the ridge. The root tapers gradually, and the root tip frequently has a mesial inclination.

Lingual Surface. The outline is the reverse of the labial view, but narrower, because the lingual converges. The structures are the same as those on the maxillary canine, but less pronounced (Figure 7-8).

Proximal Surfaces. Again, the tooth is broad from this view, with an overall shape resembling that of the maxillary canine (Figure 7-9). There are deep depressions on both the mesial and distal root surfaces.

CLINICAL CONSIDERATIONS
Root length: 16 mm
Root depressions/furrows: Deep depressions on both mesial and distal surfaces
CEJ: Curves incisally 1–2.5 mm on mesial and distal surfaces
Cervical area: No concavity on either mesial or distal surface

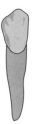
Lingual

FIGURE 7-8
Mandibular canine—lingual surface

Summary of the Mandibular Canine

Labial Surface. The characteristics of this surface are:
- A mesial cusp slope that is shorter than the distal.
- Contact areas that are more incisal than on the maxillary canine.
- A straight mesial side.
- A slightly convex distal side.
- A tapered root.

Lingual Surface. The characteristics of this surface are:
- An outline that is the reverse of the labial view, but narrower.
- Cingulum and marginal ridges that are smoother than the maxillary canine.
- Two fossae divided by the lingual ridge.
- Fossae that are shallower than on the maxillary canine.

Proximal Surfaces. The characteristics of these surfaces are:
- Greater width, providing stability.
- Deep depressions on the root surface.

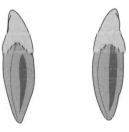
Mesial   Distal

FIGURE 7-9
Mandibular canine—mesial and distal surface

SUMMARY

Canines, along with the incisors, are considered anterior teeth. Both maxillary and mandibular canines are long, broad, pointed teeth with a sharp cusp that is used to tear food when necessary. These strong, stable teeth are located at the corners of the arch. The pronounced buccal ridge of the crown and the canine eminence of the root provide shape to the face.

WORKSHEET

A. Complete the following chart with the information requested.

	Maxillary Canine	Mandibular Canine
Universal Number		
Palmer's Notation		
Eruption Date		
Antagonists		
Anomalies		
Location of Contact Area		
Mesial		
Distal		
Succedaneous		
Number of Lobes		
*Labial Depressions**		
*Lingual**		
Ridges		
Cingulum		
Fossa		
Root Shape and Depressions		
Labial		
Proximal		

*Indicate location, size, and/or shape

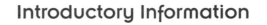

SECTION III

Permanent Posterior Teeth

Lobes

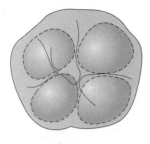

Occlusal

FIGURE III-1
The occlusal view of the maxillary first molar showing the lobes and how they come together

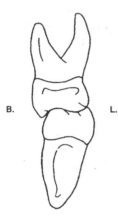

B.   L.

FIGURE III-2
Molars in occlusion—proximal view

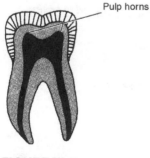

Pulp horns

FIGURE III-3
Pulp horns

INTRODUCTORY INFORMATION

After you have finished this section, you will be able to identify the location in the dental arch of each posterior tooth, as well as its universal number, expected eruption date, usual crown and root completion dates, function, lengths of crown and root, antagonists and the location of contact areas, number of lobes, and pulp canals. You will be able to state at what age there is evidence of calcification in the formation of each tooth.

You will be able to describe the location and contour of the buccal, lingual, proximal, and occlusal surfaces as they apply to each posterior tooth. Your descriptions will include contact areas, grooves, cusps, pits, ridges, fossae, outlines, contact areas, and roots of the teeth. Use Appendix D to compare the depth of the cervical lines of the teeth and to identify the location of the root depressions.

You will also be able to define terms such as **comminution**, **intercuspation**, **interdigitation**, **bifurcation**, and **marginal**, **oblique**, **transverse**, and **triangular ridges**.

To avoid redundancy in each chapter, the following descriptions consolidate information relating to posterior teeth (Figure III-1).

Related Information

Occlusal Surface. The chewing surface. All posterior teeth have a chewing surface shaped by cusps, fossae, ridges, and grooves. The lingual cusps of the maxillary teeth sit in the fossae of the mandibular teeth and vice versa (Figure III-2). Cusps slope toward the grooves so that the teeth interdigitate when in contact with each other.

Lobes. Centers of calcification. All teeth develop from at least four lobes. The premolars, with two cusps, develop from four lobes: three buccal and one lingual. The mandibular second premolar, which has three cusps, develops from five lobes: three buccal and two lingual. Lobe formation of molars is equal to the number of cusps on the tooth. If a molar has four cusps, it develops from four lobes.

Pulp Canals. The portions of the pulp located in the root of the tooth. Each root has one pulp canal *except* the mandibular first molar; the mesial root of this tooth usually has two pulp canals.

Pulp Horn. The portion in the pulp chamber, or coronal pulp, that is elevated toward a cusp (Figure III-3).

Root Trunk. The portion of the root that extends from the cemento-enamel junction to the furcation. If the root trunk divides into two roots, it is **bifurcated**. All mandibular molars have bifurcated roots. All maxillary molars are **trifurcated**—that is, divided into three roots. The area on the root trunk where it separates is called the **furcation** or forking (Figure III-4).

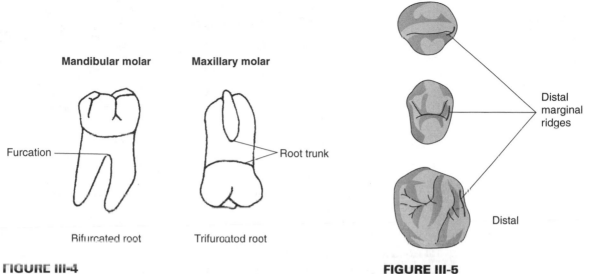

Mandibular molar   **Maxillary molar**

Furcation ———

Root trunk

Bifurcated root   Trifurcated root

Distal marginal ridges

Distal

FIGURE III-4
Furcated roots

FIGURE III-5
The marginal ridges of the maxillary central, premolar, and molar

Contact Area. The portion of the mesial or distal surface that touches, or contacts, the proximal tooth.

Succedaneous Tooth. A tooth that succeeds another tooth in the same position. Premolars are the only posterior teeth that are succedaneous. They succeed the deciduous molars. As permanent molars do not replace deciduous teeth, they are not succedaneous teeth.

Structures Common to All Posterior Teeth

Ridge. A linear elevation, named by its location or direction. There are several types:

> *Marginal ridge*: A ridge around the perimeter of the occlusal surface (Figure III-5).
> *Transverse ridge*: A ridge that crosses the occlusal surface from buccal to lingual (Figure III-6).
> *Triangular ridge*: A ridge that slants from the cusp tip toward a groove and forms a triangular slope (Figure III-7).
> *Oblique ridge*: A ridge that diagonally crosses the occlusal surface—for example, from mesio-buccal to disto-lingual (Figure III-8).
> *Cusp ridge*: A ridge that slopes from the tip of the cusp toward the mesial or distal surface.

Fossa. A shallow depression named by its shape:

> *Circular fossa*: A rounded depression.
> *Triangular fossa*: A "V"-shaped depression.
> *Irregular fossa*: A depression without definite shape.

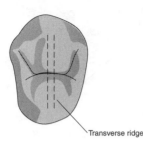

FIGURE III-6

The maxillary right first premolar occlusal surface showing the transverse ridge

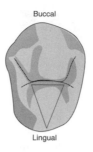

FIGURE III-7

Triangular ridge identified on the occlusal surface of a maxillary second premolar

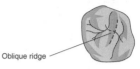

FIGURE III-8

A maxillary first molar with the oblique ridge identified

Groove. A linear depression (Figures III-9 A-E and III-10 A-D). Each posterior tooth has a primary groove pattern common to that tooth. These groove patterns are described in later chapters. Posterior teeth usually have additional or supplementary grooves that are not included with the descriptions or in the illustrations because of their variation in each person.

Pit. A pinpoint depression where two or more grooves meet (Figure III-11).

Facts to Help Avoid Confusion

Premolars. Since these teeth usually have two cusps, they are alternately referred to as bicuspids. However, the mandibular second premolar

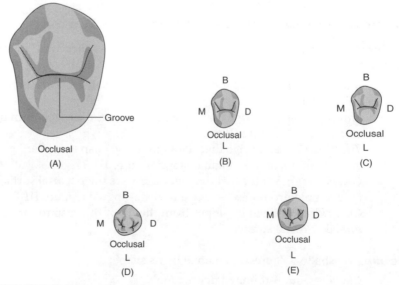

FIGURE III-9 A-E

(A) A groove on the occlusal surface of a maxillary first premolar where the lobes were united. (B)–(E) Occlusal surfaces of the maxillary and mandibular premolars

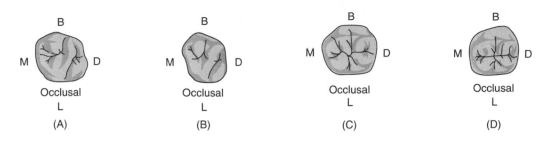

FIGURE III-10 A-D
Occlusal surfaces of the maxillary and mandibular molars

often has three cusps; therefore, these teeth are more accurately called pre-molars. All premolars have a well-developed middle buccal lobe that forms a buccal ridge ending at a pointed cusp.

Nomenclature. Cusps, grooves, fossae, and ridges are commonly named by their location, such as mesio-buccal cusp, central groove, or distal marginal ridge (Figure III-12). With a little thought, you can probably name most of the structures without having to memorize them. Note that when the words "mesial" or "distal" are used in combination with another surface, the "al" is changed to "o" as in "mesiolingual."

Size and Shape of Surfaces. Because the mouth has less space toward the posterior region, distal surfaces of the teeth are generally smaller than mesial structures. Crowns, too, tip distally so that more of the occlusal surface can be seen when the distal side of the tooth is viewed.

Occlusal surface. Technically, the occlusal surface is within the borders of the cusp and marginal ridges. However, when the occlusal surface is described in the following chapters, all structures, seen from this view, are noted.

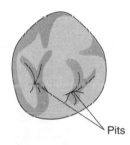

FIGURE III-11
The pits of a mandibular first premolar on the occlusal surface

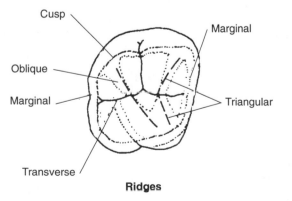

FIGURE III-12
Maxillary first molar—occlusal surface

Maxillary Premolars

KEY TERMS

Root trunk

Bifurcated

Buccal ridge

Mesial concavity

Mesial interradicular groove

Triangular ridge

Triangular fossa

Major groove pattern

OBJECTIVES

- Identify the maxillary premolars and provide vital information: that is, universal number, function, antagonists, and so forth.
- Describe the location and contour of each maxillary premolar.
- Define the new terms in the chapter.
- Complete the worksheet at the end of the chapter.

GENERAL INFORMATION

There are four maxillary premolars: two in each quadrant. They are named by their position in the arch from anterior to posterior as first premolar and second premolar.

Maxillary premolars have one buccal and one lingual cusp. Both premolars have a prominent middle buccal lobe extending from the cervix to the tip of the buccal cusp, similar to the canine, with shallow depressions on either side.

The **root trunk** of the maxillary first premolar is **bifurcated**, dividing into two roots (buccal and lingual) that are seen only from the proximal view. The maxillary second premolar has only one root.

Viewed from the buccal, all premolars resemble one another, with their pointed buccal cusp and tapered root, so it is difficult to differentiate them. However, each has a unique structure on another surface that will assist in its identification.

Premolars replace deciduous molars; there are no deciduous premolars. The first premolar succeeds the deciduous first molar; the second premolar succeeds the deciduous second molar.

With their triangular-shaped cusps and fossae, the premolars are structured to assist with the grinding of food.

MAXILLARY FIRST PREMOLAR

Characteristics

Location in the Arch	Fourth tooth from the midline; distal to cuspid
Universal Number	R-#5 L-#12
Eruption Date	10–11 years
First Evidence of Calcification	$1\frac{1}{2}$ years
Crown Completion	5–6 years
Root Completion	12–13 years
Function	Grinding
Length of Crown	8.5 mm
Length of Root	14 mm
Antagonists	Mandibular first and second premolar

Location of Contact Area

Mesial	Middle of the tooth
Distal	Slightly more occlusal than the mesial contact

Identifying Features

- two cusps: one buccal, one lingual
- two roots: one buccal, one lingual
- two pulp canals: one in each root
- resembles canine but is shorter
- mesial marginal groove

- mesial concavity around CEJ
- mesial root depression (mesial inter radicular groove) from CEJ to furcation

(Refer to Figure 8-1)

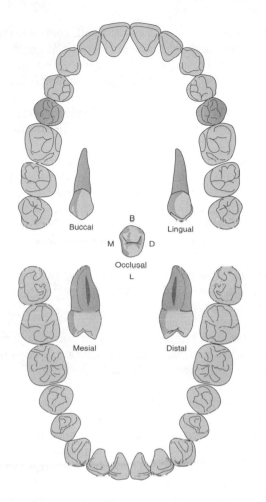

B
Buccal   Lingual
M   D
Occlusal
L

Mesial   Distal

FIGURE 8-1
Maxillary first premolars

Tooth Description of the Maxillary First Premolar

Buccal Surface. Only the buccal cusp and buccal root are visible, obscuring the shorter lingual cusp and root positioned directly behind them. A well-developed middle buccal lobe forms a **buccal ridge** extending from the cervix to the tip of the pointed buccal cusp (Figure 8-2). Shallow depressions parallel the ridge. The mesial cusp slope is longer than the distal cusp slope.

The *mesial side* is concave from the cervix to the contact area at the middle of the surface. The *distal side* is straighter than the mesial from the cervix to the contact area. The distal contact area is slightly more occlusal than the mesial, making the distal cusp slope shorter. The buccal root is tapered.

Lingual Surface. Both cusps are visible from this view (Figure 8-3). As the lingual cusp is approximately 1 mm shorter, the tip of the buccal cusp extends below it. The lingual cusp is smooth—no ridge, no depressions. Some of the mesial and distal surfaces of both the crown and the root are seen because the lingual surface is narrower than the buccal.

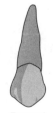

Buccal

FIGURE 8-2
Maxillary first premolar—buccal surface

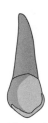

Lingual

FIGURE 8-3

Maxillary first premolar—
lingual surface

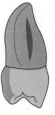

Mesial   **Distal**

FIGURE 8-4

Maxillary second premolar—
mesial and distal surfaces

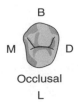

B

M   D

Occlusal

L

FIGURE 8-5

Maxillary first premolar—
occlusal surface

Proximal Surfaces. Both cusps and both roots are visible. Although the tooth appears small from the buccal view, it is about 2 mm wider when viewed from the proximal surface, from buccal to lingual. Both cusps are within the confines of the roots, thus helping to absorb some of the pressure from mastication.

The root trunk is bifurcated for one-half or less of its length. Both roots are straight until the apical third, where they incline toward each other.

Mesial Surface. Extending from the occlusal surface and crossing the marginal ridge onto the mesial surface is a mesial marginal groove (Figure 8-4). At its end, only a sort distance onto the mesial surface, is a **mesial concavity** that continues onto the root and merges with the root bifurcation. There is a deep groove on the root that extends from the CEJ to bifurcation. It is termed the **mesial interradicular groove**.

Distal Surface. The distal surface of the crown is smooth; it has no groove or depression. The root does have a depression that extends into the bifurcation (Figure 8-4).

Occlusal Surface. The occlusal shape forms a hexagon, circumscribed by the marginal and cusp ridges. Because the cusps tip inward, both the buccal and lingual surfaces are visible (Figure 8-5).

Note that the buccal cusp tip is centered between the mesial and distal sides (Figure 8-6). Both the buccal and lingual cusps are pyramid shaped, with their sides sloping toward the central groove and fossae. The slope from the tip of the buccal cusp to the central groove and from the tip of the lingual cusp to the central groove, forms a **triangular ridge**. The two fossae are the mesial triangular fossa and the distal **triangular fossa**.

Located at the base of the cusps, and separating them, are the grooves. Although there can be several supplementary grooves, the **major groove pattern** common to all maxillary first premolars includes the central, mesiobuccal, distobuccal, mesial marginal, and distolingual grooves (Figure 8-6). As with most occlusal patterns, these structures are named by their location.

It is common to find a pit where two or more grooves merge. Thus, it is likely that this occlusal will have a mesial and distal pit located in the fossae.

CLINICAL CONSIDERATIONS

Root length: 14 mm

Root depressions/furrows: Deep depression on mesial surface extending from crown to root furcation, where there is a deeper groove into the bifurcation. Length of root trunk is approximately 7 mm from cervix to bifurcation. Distal root trunk has a depression extending from cervix to bifurcation.

CEJ: Very slight curvature (0–1 mm toward occlusal) on both mesial and distal surfaces.

Cervical area: Concave on both mesial and distal surfaces, with deeper concavity on the mesial surface.

Furcation: Approximately 7 mm from cervix

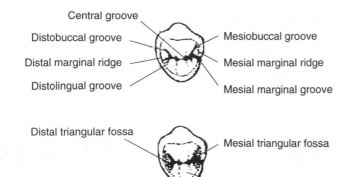

FIGURE 8-6

Maxillary first premolar—occlusal surface

Summary of the Maxillary First Premolar

Buccal Surface.   The characteristics of this surface are:

- A prominent buccal ridge.
- A pointed buccal cusp.
- A mesial side that is concave from the cervix to the contact area; a contact area that is in the middle of the surface; a cusp slope that is straighter and longer than the distal.
- A distal side that is straight from the cervix to the contact area; a contact area that is more occlusal than on the mesial; a cusp slope that is shorter than the mesial.
- Only the buccal root is visible.

Lingual Surface.   The characteristics of this surface are:

- Both cusps are visible.
- A smooth lingual cusp that is shorter and narrower than the buccal cusp.
- Visible mesial and distal surfaces.

Proximal Surfaces.   The characteristics of these surfaces are:

- Two visible cusps; a lingual cusp that is 1 mm shorter than the buccal cusp.
- Two visible roots (two pulp canals).
- Cusps that are within the confines of the root trunk.
- A mesial crown surface with the mesial marginal groove and a mesial concavity that extends from the crown to the root bifurcation.
- A distal crown surface with no grooves and no depressions.
- Both roots straight until the apical third, then incline toward each other.
- Root that bifurcates for one-half its length with a deep mesial interradicular groove.

Occlusal Surface.   The characteristics of this surface are:
- Visible buccal and lingual surfaces.
- A buccal cusp centered between the mesial and distal side.
- Fossae: mesial and distal triangular.
- Grooves: central, mesiobuccal, mesiomarginal, distobuccal, and distolingual.

MAXILLARY SECOND PREMOLAR

Characteristics

Location in the Arch	Fifth tooth from the midline; distal to the first premolar
Universal Number.	R-#4 L-#13
Eruption Date	10–12 years
First Evidence of Calcification	2 years
Crown Completion	6–7 years
Root Completion	12–14 years
Function	Grinding
Length of Crown	8.5 mm
Length of Root	14 mm
Antagonists	Mandibular second premolar and first molar

Location of Contact Area

Mesial	Middle of the tooth
Distal	Middle of the tooth

Identifying Features
- two cusps: one buccal, one lingual
- one root, one pulp canal
- resembles first premolar with slight variations

(Refer to Figure 8-7)

Tooth Description of the Maxillary Second Premolar

The maxillary second premolar (Figure 8-8) looks like the maxillary first premolar but has the following variations:
- There is only one root and one pulp canal.
- The mesial buccal cusp slope is shorter than the distal buccal cusp slope.
- Both cusps are about the same length (lingual is slightly shorter).
- The mesial surface of the crown has no groove and no concavity. From the occlusal view, there may be a mesial marginal groove but it seldom extends onto the mesial surface.
- A shallow depression is evident on the mesial surface of the root.

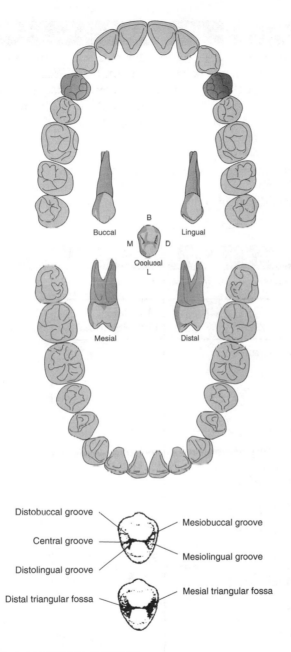

Buccal

Lingual

B

M   D

Ooolual
L

Mesial

Distal

FIGURE 8-7
Maxillary second premolars

Distobuccal groove

Central groove

Distolingual groove

Distal triangular fossa

Mesiobuccal groove

Mesiolingual groove

Mesial triangular fossa

FIGURE 8-8
Maxillary second premolar—
grooves and fossae

CLINICAL CONSIDERATIONS

Root length: 14 mm

Root depressions/furrows: A shallow depression on both mesial and distal surfaces extending the length of the root

CEJ: Very slight curvature (0–1 mm toward occlusal) on both mesial and distal surfaces

Cervical area: Concave on both mesial and distal surfaces, with deeper concavity on the mesial surface

Furcation: None

SUMMARY

Maxillary premolars are positioned just distal to the maxillary canines. There are two in each maxillary quadrant. Each premolar has two cusps, a buccal and a lingual, which account for their alternate designation of bicuspids. Lying between the cusps is an occlusal surface, which is used to crush and grind the food in preparation for digestion.

Premolars replace deciduous molars. These teeth, along with the molars, are considered posterior teeth.

The maxillary first premolar has two roots and two pulp canals; the second premolar has only one. Because of their similarities, the roots are the easiest way to distinguish the first from the second premolar.

WORKSHEET

Complete the following chart with the information requested.

	Maxillary First Premolar	Maxillary Second Premolar
Universal Number		
Palmer's Notation		
Eruption Date		
Antagonists		
Succedaneous		
Number of Cusps		
Number of Roots		
Identifying Features*		
Buccal		
Lingual		
Mesial		
Distal		
Occlusal Description		
Cusps		
Fossae		
Grooves		

*Size, number of cusps, location of grooves, etc.

Mandibular Premolars

KEY TERMS

Buccal ridge

Nonfunctioning cusp

Mesiolingual groove

Transverse ridge

Y-shaped groove pattern

OBJECTIVES

- Identify the mandibular premolars and provide vital information: that is, universal number, function, antagonist, and so forth.
- Describe the location and contour of each mandibular premolar.
- Define the new terms in the chapter.
- Complete the worksheet at the end of the chapter.

GENERAL INFORMATION

There are four mandibular premolars: two in each quadrant. They are named by their position in the arch from anterior to posterior as first premolar and second premolar.

The mandibular first premolar has one buccal and one lingual cusp. Differing from the others, the mandibular second premolar often has one buccal and two lingual cusps; it is the only premolar with three cusps.

Both mandibular premolars usually have one root. Mandibular premolars assist the maxillary premolars with grinding and chewing food.

MANDIBULAR FIRST PREMOLAR

Characteristics
Location in the Arch . . . . Fourth tooth from the midline; distal to canine
Universal Number . . . . R-#28   L-#21
Eruption Date . . . . 10–12 years
First Evidence of Calcification . . . . . $1\frac{1}{4}$–2 years
Crown Completion . . . . 5–6 years
Root Completion . . . . 12–13 years
Function . . . . Grinding
Length of Crown . . . . 8.5 mm
Length of Root . . . . 14 mm
Antagonists . . . . Maxillary cuspid and first premolar

Location of Contact Area
Mesial . . . . Middle of the tooth
Distal . . . . Middle of the tooth

Identifying Features
• two cusps: one buccal, one lingual
• lingual cusp is small and nonfunctioning
• one root, which sometimes tends to bifurcate at the apex
• mesiolingual groove

(Refer to Figure 9-1)

Tooth Description of the Mandibular First Premolar

Buccal Surface.   A very prominent **buccal ridge**, perhaps more rounded than any of the other premolars, extends to a pointed cusp (Figure 9-2). Again, as was evident in the maxillary premolars, shallow depression occurs on either side of the buccal ridge. The mesial cusp slope is shorter than the distal.

The *mesial side* is concave from the cervix to the rounded contact area in the middle of the surface. The *distal* outline is also slightly concave from the cervix to the contact area, at about the middle of the tooth.

The cervix is narrow. The root is tapered and about 3–4 mm shorter than the adjacent cuspid.

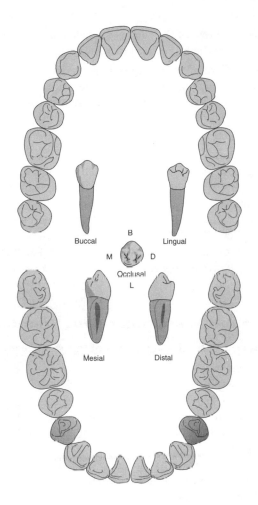

FIGURE 9-1
Mandibular first premolars

Lingual Surface. The lingual cusp is short and poorly developed, extending only two-thirds the height of the crown (Figure 9-3). It is a **non-functioning cusp**. Because of the position of the cusps, most of the occlusal surface can be seen from this view. Extending from the occlusal surface onto the lingual is a **mesiolingual groove** that delineates the lingual cusp.

Mesial Surface.   Both the buccal and lingual cusps, as well as some of the occlusal surface, are seen (Figure 9-4). The tip of the buccal cusp is centered over the root. Parallel to the buccal triangular ridge is the mesial marginal ridge, which is interrupted, or broken, by the mesiolingual groove.

A broad root, tapering only at the apical third, has a deep developmental groove near the apex. Often this groove will bifurcate the tip of the root.

Distal Surface.   The overall shape is the reverse of the mesial, but the surface structures vary. The distal marginal ridge is perpendicular to the buccal cusp ridge, and there is no interruption by grooves (Figure 9-4). The root has a shallow depression, but there is seldom a groove near the apical third.

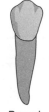

Buccal

FIGURE 9-2
Mandibular first premolar—
buccal surface

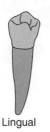

FIGURE 9-3
Mandibular first premolar—
lingual surface

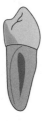
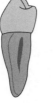

FIGURE 9-4
Mandibular first premolar—
mesial and distal surfaces

Occlusal View.   Most of the buccal surface can be seen from this view (Figure 9-5), as well as the following occlusal structures:

- Fossae (both irregular in shape): mesial, distal
- Grooves: mesiobuccal, distobuccal, mesiolingual
- **Transverse ridge**: connects the buccal and lingual cusps

CLINICAL CONSIDERATIONS
Root length: 14 mm
Root depressions/furrows: Mesial depression becomes a deep groove near the apical third. This groove often bifurcates the root tip. The distal surface has a shallow depression but no groove at the apical third.
CEJ: Very slight curvature (0–1 mm toward occlusal) on both mesial and distal surfaces
Cervical area: Concave on both mesial and distal surfaces, with deeper concavity on the mesial surface
Furcation: None

Summary of the Mandibular First Premolar

Buccal Surface.   The characteristics of this surface are:

- A prominent buccal ridge.
- A pointed cusp.
- A narrow cervix.
- A mesial side that is concave from the cervix to the contact area; a contact area at the middle of the tooth; a mesial cusp slope shorter than the distal.
- A distal that is concave from the cervix to the contact area; a contact area that is in the middle of the tooth; a cusp slope that is longer than the mesial.

Lingual Surface.   The characteristics of this surface are:

- Visible mesial and distal surfaces.
- A short lingual cusp that is two-thirds the height of the crown.
- A lingual cusp that is nonfunctional.
- A mesiolingual groove that delineates the lingual cusp.

Proximal Surfaces.   The characteristics of this surface are:

- Both cusps visible.
- The tip of the buccal cusp centered over the root.

Mesiobuccal groove — Distobuccal groove

Mesiolingual groove

FIGURE 9-5
Mandibular first premolar—
occlusal surface

Mesial (irregular) fossa — Distal (irregular) fossa

- A visible occlusal surface.
- A mesial surface with a mesiomarginal ridge that is parallel to the buccal triangular ridge; a mesiolingual groove that interrupts the mesiomarginal ridge; a slight curve in the cervical line; a broad root with a deep developmental groove at the apical third.
- A distal surface with a distal marginal ridge that is perpendicular to the buccal cusp ridge; a marginal ridge that is uninterrupted; a root that has a shallow depression but seldom has a groove; a cervical line that is straight; a concavity on the surface near the cervical line.

Occlusal Surface. The characteristics of this surface are:

- A visible buccal surface.
- Two irregular fossae: mesial and distal.
- Grooves: mesiobuccal, distobuccal, and mesiolingual.
- A prominent transverse ridge.

MANDIBULAR SECOND PREMOLAR

Characteristics

Location in the Arch	Fifth tooth from the midline; distal to the first premolar
Universal Number	R-#29 L-#20
Eruption Date	11–12 years
First Evidence of Calcification	2$\frac{1}{2}$ years
Crown Completion	6–7 years
Root Completion	13–14 years
Function	Grinding
Length of Crown	8 mm
Length of Root	14.5 mm
Antagonists	Maxillary first and second premolar

Location of Contact Area

Mesial	Middle of the tooth
Distal	Middle of the tooth

Identifying Features

- three cusps: buccal, mesiolingual, distolingual
- one root, one pulp canal

(Refer to Figure 9-6)

Tooth Description of the Mandibular Second Premolar

The following description is of a mandibular second premolar with three cusps: the buccal, mesiolingual, and distolingual. When the mandibular second premolar has only two cusps, it resembles the mandibular first premolar.

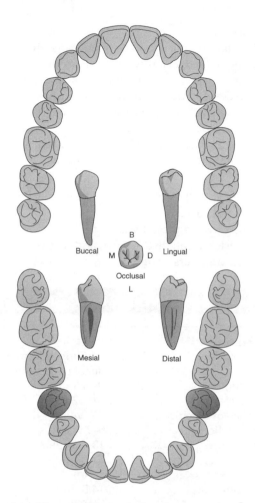

FIGURE 9-6
Mandibular second premolars

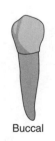

Buccal

FIGURE 9-7
Mandibular second
premolar—buccal surface

Buccal Surface. From the buccal view the second premolar looks similar to the first premolar, but it is slightly broader and shorter with contact areas a bit more occlusal than the first premolar. Only the buccal cusp is visible (Figure 9-7).

Lingual Surface. Because the lingual cusps are shorter than the buccal cusp, all three cusps are visible from this aspect. Both the mesiolingual and the distolingual cusps are functioning cusps. Separating the two lingual cusps is the lingual groove (Figure 9-8). The mesiolingual cusp is the larger of the two lingual cusps.

Mesial Surface. Because the mesial side of the tooth is larger than the distal, only the buccal and mesiolingual cusps are visible (Figure 9-9). The mesial marginal ridge forms a right angle with the buccal cusp slope; it is not broken by a groove. The mesial surface is smooth, with only a slight curvature at the cervical line. The root is broad, tapering at the apical third.

Distal Surface. Because the teeth converge toward the posterior portion of the mouth, the distal of the tooth is narrower than the mesial, revealing some of the occlusal surface. All three cusps can be seen (Figure 9-9).

Occlusal Surface. The order of cusp size, from largest to smallest, is buccal, mesiolingual, and distolingual. The cusps are divided by grooves forming a **"Y"-shaped groove pattern** (Figure 9-10). There are two fossae, both triangular in shape: mesial and distal triangular fossae. There is no transverse ridge on the three cusp variety. There would be a transverse ridge on the two cusp premolar.

CLINICAL CONSIDERATIONS
Root length: 14.5 mm
Root depressions/furrows: Generally smooth, but mesial may have a shallow depression
CEJ: Very slight curvature (0–1 mm toward occlusal) on both mesial and distal surfaces
Cervical area: Slightly concave on both mesial and distal surfaces
Furcation: None

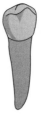

Lingual

FIGURE 9-8
Mandibular second premolar—lingual surface

Summary of the Mandibular Second Premolar

Buccal Surface. The characteristics of this surface are:

- A resemblance to the mandibular first premolar but slightly shorter and broader.
- Contact areas are in the middle of the tooth but slightly more occlusal than in the first premolar.

Lingual Surface. The characteristics of this surface are:

- Three visible cusps: buccal, mesiolingual, and distolingual.
- Cusps are all functioning.
- Lingual cusps are shorter than the buccal cusp.
- A lingual groove that divides the two lingual cusps.

Proximal Surfaces. The characteristics of these surfaces are:

- A mesial surface with visible buccal and mesiolingual cusps; a mesial marginal ridge that forms a right angle with the buccal cusp slope; a cervical line that has a slight curvature.
- A distal surface having more of the occlusal surface visible; all three cusps visible.
- Cusps, which in order of size are buccal, mesiolingual, and distolingual.
- A broad root tapering at the apical third.

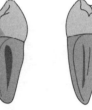

Mesial   Distal

FIGURE 9-9
Mandibular second premolar— mesial and distal surfaces

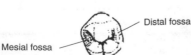

Mesiobuccal groove
Distobuccal groove
Lingual groove

Distal fossa
Mesial fossa

FIGURE 9-10
Mandibular second premolar—occlusal surface

Occlusal Surface. The characteristics of this surface are:

- Two triangular fossae: mesial and distal.
- Mesiobuccal, distobuccal, and lingual grooves.
- Grooves that form a "Y" shape on a three cusp tooth.

SUMMARY

Mandibular premolars are positioned just distal to the mandibular canines. There are two in each mandibular quadrant. Although the first premolar has two cusps, the second premolar frequently has three cusps; consequently, the term "bicuspid" would not be appropriate for this tooth.

The mandibular first premolar has not only a sharp, pointed buccal cusp but also a short, nonfunctioning lingual cusp that makes this tooth easy to distinguish from other premolars. The mandibular second premolar may have two cusps and resemble the first, but it frequently has three cusps (one buccal and two lingual) that are nearly the same height.

As with all posterior teeth, the occlusal surface is located between the cusps and outlined by marginal ridges. All cusps slope into grooves located at the base of the occlusal surface.

WORKSHEET

A. Complete the following chart with the information requested.

	Mandibular First Premolar	Mandibular Second Premolar
Universal Number		
Palmer's Notation		
Eruption Date		
Antagonists		
Succedaneous		
Number of Cusps		
Number of Roots		
Identifying Features*		
Buccal		
Lingual		
Mesial		
Distal		
Occlusal Description		
Cusps		
Fossae		
Grooves		

*Size, number of cusps, location of grooves, etc.

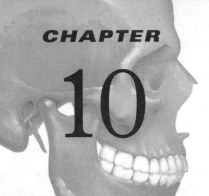

Maxillary First and Second Molars

KEY TERMS

Tuborolc

Cusp of Carabelli

Trifurcated

Pulp canal

Oblique ridge

Succedaneous

OBJECTIVES

- Identify the maxillary first and second molars and provide vital information: that is, universal number, function, antagonist, and so forth.
- Describe the location and contour of each first and second maxillary molar.
- Define the new terms in the chapter.
- Complete the worksheet at the end of the chapter.

GENERAL INFORMATION

There are six maxillary molars: three in each quadrant. Like the premolars, molars are named by their position in the arch from anterior to posterior or first molar, second molar, and third molar. Permanent molars erupt posterior to the primary second molars and do not replace deciduous teeth.

The first molar is the first permanent tooth to erupt. The mandibular first molar precedes the maxillary first molar by a few months, but both usually erupt before the permanent central incisors.

With the exception of third molars, all maxillary molars have at least four cusps. The maxillary first molar usually has a fifth, nonfunctioning cusp, or **tubercle**, that is positioned on another cusp. This fifth cusp is known as the **cusp of Carabelli**. The number of lobes from which a molar develops is the same as the number of cusps.

Maxillary molars have **trifurcated** (divided into three) roots: mesiobuccal, distobuccal, and lingual. Each root has one **pulp canal**.

Molars are structured so that they are narrower (that is, they converge) toward the posterior portion of the mouth. Thus, the distal of the tooth is narrower than the mesial. Because they have multicusps, molars perform the major tasks of mastication and comminution by grinding and pulverizing food.

MAXILLARY FIRST MOLAR

Characteristics

Location in the Arch	Sixth tooth from the midline; distal to maxillary second pre-molar
Universal Number	R-#3 L-#14
Eruption Date	6–7 years
First Evidence of Calcification	Birth
Crown Completion	2$\frac{1}{2}$–3 years
Root Completion	9–10 years
Function	Mastication and comminution of food
Length of Crown	7.5 mm
Length of Root	12 mm buccal 13 mm lingual
Antagonists	Mandibular first and second molars

Location of Contact Area

Mesial	2/3 distance from cervical line
Distal	Middle of the tooth

Identifying Features

- five cusps: mesiobuccal, distobuccal, mesiolingual, distolingual, cusp of Carabelli

(continues)

MAXILLARY FIRST MOLAR (continued)

- three roots: mesiobuccal, distobuccal, lingual
- three pulp canals, one in each root, the mesiobuccal root may have two pulp canals
- cusp of Carabelli, or fifth cusp, located on the mesiolingual cusp, is a nonfunctioning cusp
- largest and strongest of the maxillary teeth

(Refer to Figure 10-1)

Tooth Description of the Maxillary First Molar

Buccal Surface. The two buccal cusps and the cusp tips of the two longer lingual cusps are seen from this view (Figure 10-2). Dividing the mesiobuccal and distobuccal cusps is the buccal groove. This extends about one-half the length of the crown, ending in a shallow depression.

The mesial side, from cervix to contact area, is straight. The contact area, located about two-thirds the distance from the cervical line, is convex.

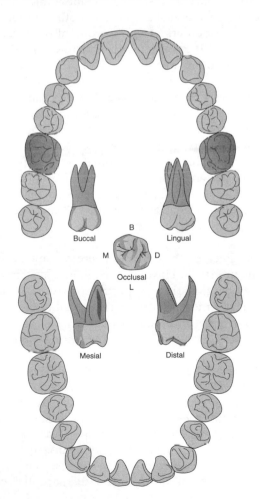

Buccal　B　Lingual

M　D

Occlusal
L

Mesial　Distal

FIGURE 10-1

Maxillary first molars

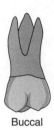

FIGURE 10-2
Maxillary first molar—buccal surface

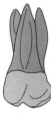

FIGURE 10-3
Maxillary first molar—lingual surface

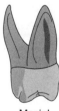

FIGURE 10-4
Maxillary first molar—mesial surface

The distal side is convex and reaches the contact area in the middle of the tooth. The cervical line forms a slight curve.

Before bifurcating into the mesiobuccal and distobuccal root, the root trunk extends about 4 mm. A shallow depression continues from the cervical line to its end as a deep groove at the bifurcation. The mesiobuccal root extends halfway in a mesial direction before curving distally; the smaller distobuccal root is straight for half its length, then curves mesially. The mesiobuccal root may have two pulp canals. Seen between the two buccal roots and extending above them by 1 mm is the lingual root.

Lingual Surface.   As the two lingual cusps, mesiolingual and distolingual, are longer than the buccal cusps, they block the buccal cusps from view. Dividing the two lingual cusps is the lingual groove (Figure 10-3). The mesiolingual cusp is about three-fifths the width of the crown and supports the fifth cusp, **the cusp (or tubercle) of Carabelli.** The mesiolingual cusp is the largest cusp. The fifth cusp is not always present; even when it is, it may not be well-developed as it is a nonfunctioning cusp. A short groove, the fifth cusp groove, is usually present on the mesiolingual cusp when the tubercle is absent. The distolingual cusp is a smooth spheroid.

Although the lateral borders of the two buccal roots can be seen, the lingual root is dominant. It is broad with a furrow extending most of its length, and it tapers to a blunt apex.

Mesial Surface.   Because the mesial side is wider than the distal, only the mesiobuccal and mesiolingual cusps and the cusp of Carabelli are seen. The mesial marginal ridge, connecting the cusps, is about one-fifth the distance from the cusp tips; it obstructs the occlusal surface. Just cervical to the contact area is a shallow depression that continues from the crown onto the root trunk.

Both the mesiobuccal and lingual root block the smaller distal root. The mesiobuccal root is flat but broad, with a depression spanning most of its length. The lingual root is long and narrow (banana-shaped) from this aspect (Figure 10-4).

Distal Surface.   Because the crown converges, some of the buccal surface can be seen (Figure 10-5). The distal marginal ridge curves more cervically than the mesial marginal ridge, exposing some of the occlusal surface.

The cervical line is almost straight. Although all three roots are visible, only the outline of the mesiobuccal root can be seen. From the cervical line to the distobuccal root is a depression. There is no concavity at the bifurcation.

Occlusal Surface.   The width from buccal to lingual is wider than from mesial to distal. Looking down onto the occlusal surface, you can more easily see the convergence of the crown toward the distal and the size of the five cusps. From largest to smallest, the cusps are mesiolingual, mesiobuccal, distobuccal, distolingual, and cusp of Carabelli.

The buccal groove extends from the buccal surface onto the occlusal and joins the central groove (Figure 10-6). The distobuccal cusp and the mesiolingual cusp, which form an **oblique ridge**, are divided by a transverse groove, an extension of the central groove that continues into the distal fossa. On the occlusal surface, the two lingual cusps are divided by the distal oblique groove, an extension of the lingual groove (lingual surface) that, obviously, extends obliquely into the distal fossa.

All cusps slope downward toward the grooves. It is the base and sides of the cusp slopes that form the fossa. On this tooth there is a large circular central fossa. Notice, in Figure 10-6, the number of cusps that slope into it. The two lingual cusps slope into the distal linear fossa as well as into the mesial and distal triangular fossa.

CLINICAL CONSIDERATIONS

Root length: Buccal is 12 mm; lingual is 13 mm.

Root depressions: (1) On the buccal surface, a shallow depression from cervical line ends in a deep groove at the bifurcation. Root trunk is approximately 4 mm in length. (2) On the lingual surface, a broad depression extends most of its length. (3) On the mesial surface, a depression from the contact area of the crown continues onto the root trunk; the mesiobuccal root has a broad depression extending most of its length; and the lingual root is smooth. Bifurcation is approximately 4 mm from cervix. (4) On the distal surface, a depression extends from the cervical line to the distobuccal root. Root bifurcation occurs at 4–5 mm, with no concavity.

CEJ: Very slight curvature (0–1 mm toward occlusal) on both mesial and distal surfaces

Cervical area from buccal or lingual surface: Both the mesial and distal surfaces are concave

Distal

FIGURE 10-5

Maxillary first molar—distal surface

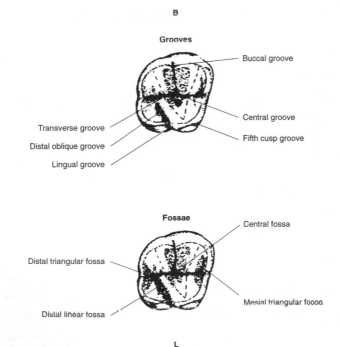

B

Grooves

— Buccal groove

— Central groove

Transverse groove —

Distal oblique groove —

Lingual groove —

— Fifth cusp groove

Fossae

— Central fossa

Distal triangular fossa —

Mesial triangular fossa

Distal linear fossa —

L

FIGURE 10-6

Maxillary first molar— occlusal surface

Furcation: Buccal surface bifurcates at 4 mm from cervical line; mesial surface bifurcates 4 mm from cervical line; distal surface bifurcates 4–5 mm from cervical line; lingual surface, no furcation.

Summary of the Maxillary First Molar

Buccal Surface.   The characteristics of this surface are:

Crown

- Two buccal cusps: mesiobuccal and distobuccal.
- Two longer lingual cusp tips are visible.
- The buccal groove divides the two buccal cusps; it extends one-half the crown length and terminates in a shallow depression.
- The mesial outline is straight.
- The mesial contact is two-thirds the distance from the cervical line.
- The distal side is convex.
- The distal contact area is in the middle of the surface.

Root

- Two buccal roots: mesiobuccal and distobuccal.
- The mesiobuccal root extends in a mesial direction for half its length and then curves distally.
- The distobuccal root is straight for half its length, then curves mesially.
- The root trunk is about 4 mm long before bifurcating.
- A shallow depression extends from the cervical line and terminates in a deep groove at the bifurcation.
- The lingual root extends between and above the buccal roots.

Lingual Surface.   The characteristics of this surface are:

Crown

- Three visible cusps: mesiolingual, distolingual, and cusp of Carabelli.
- A mesiolingual cusp about three-fifths the width of the crown.
- A cusp of Carabelli positioned on the mesiolingual cusp.
- A fifth cusp groove on the mesiolingual cusp if the fifth cusp is not present.
- A lingual groove dividing the two lingual cusps.

Roots

- A broad, tapered lingual root, the longest of the three roots, with a furrow or depression.
- A visible outline of both buccal roots.

Mesial Surface.   The characteristics of this surface are:

Crown

- Visible cusps: mesiobuccal, mesiolingual, and cusp of Carabelli.
- A depression on the crown from the contact area to the root trunk.
- A mesial marginal ridge about one-fifth the distance from the cusp tips.

Root

- Two visible roots: a broad, flat mesiobuccal root and a tapered lingual root.
- A depression on the lingual root.

Distal Surface. The characteristics of this surface are:

Crown

- Visible buccal and occlusal surfaces.
- An almost straight cervical line.

Root

- All three roots visible (only the border of the mesiobuccal root can be seen).
- A depression from the cervical line to the distobuccal root.
- No concavity in the root bifurcation.

Occlusal Surface. The characteristics of this surface are:
- Dimensions that are wider from the buccal to the lingual than from the mesial to the distal.
- Four functioning *cusps* and a small fifth cusp (in order of size): mesiolingual, mesiobuccal, distobuccal, distolingual, and cusp of Carabelli.
- Grooves: buccal, central, transverse groove of the oblique ridge, and distal oblique; the lingual and fifth cusp groove are visible from this view.
- Fossae: central, distal linear, mesial triangular, and distal triangular.

MAXILLARY SECOND MOLAR

Characteristics

Location in the Arch	Seventh tooth from the midline; distal to the first molar
Universal Number	R-#2 L-#15
Eruption Date	12–13 years
First Evidence of Calcification	$2^1/_2$–3 years
Crown Completion	7–8 years
Root Completion	14–16 years
Function	Mastication and comminution
Length of Crown	7 mm
Length of Root	11 mm buccal 12 mm lingual
Antagonists	Mandibular second and third molars

Location of Contact Area

Mesial	2/3 from cervical line
Distal	Middle of the tooth

(continues)

MAXILLARY SECOND MOLAR (continued)

Identifying Features
- four cusps: mesiobuccal, distobuccal, mesiolingual, distolingual
- three roots: mesiobuccal, distobuccal, lingual
- three pulp canals—one in each root

(Refer to Figure 10-7)

Tooth Description of the Maxillary Second Molar

The maxillary second molar is similar to the maxillary first molar in size, shape, and function but has the following differences:

- Both crown and root are slightly smaller.
- The second molar has only four cusps: mesiobuccal, distobuccal, mesiolingual, and distolingual.
- There is no cusp of Carabelli.

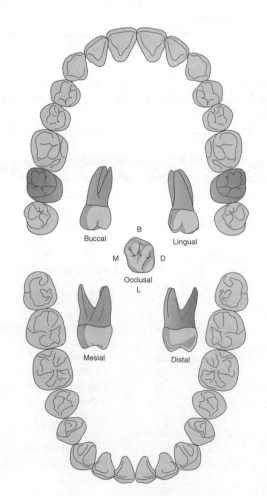

FIGURE 10-7
Maxillary second molars

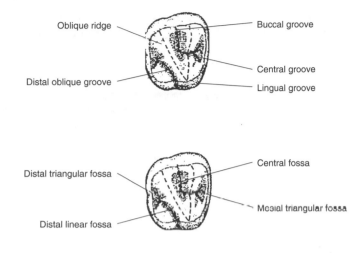

FIGURE 10-8
Maxillary second molar—occlusal surface

- The roots are not as divergent. They are closer together.
- The occlusal surface has more supplementary grooves.
- There is no transverse groove of the oblique ridge.

Occlusal Surface.   The characteristics of this surface, shown in Figure 10-8, are:

- Grooves: buccal, lingual, distal oblique, and central groove
- Fossae: central, distal linear, distal triangular, and mesial triangular
- Cusps, in order of size: mesiolingual, mesiobuccal, distobuccal, and distolingual

CLINICAL CONSIDERATIONS
Root length: 11 mm buccal; 12 mm lingual
Root depressions/furrows: Similar to those on maxillary first molar
CEJ: Very slight curvature (0–1 mm toward occlusal) on mesial and distal surfaces
Cervical area from buccal or lingual surface: Similar to that of maxillary first molar
Furcation: Similar to that of maxillary first molar

SUMMARY

There are three maxillary molars in each maxillary quadrant. They have at least four cusps and a broad occlusal surface. Because of their size, the molars perform the major task of grinding and pulverizing food.

The maxillary first molar has four functioning cusps and one small tubercle on the mesiolingual cusp called the fifth cusp, or cusp of Carabelli. The first molar is the largest and strongest of the maxillary teeth. The second molar resembles the first but does not have a fifth cusp, and its overall dimensions are slightly smaller than the first.

All maxillary molars have three roots, each with one pulp canal. The mesiobuccal root of the maxillary first molar may have two pulp canals. Molars are *not* **succedaneous** teeth.

WORKSHEET

A. Complete the following chart with the information requested.

	Maxillary First Molar	Maxillary Second Molar
Universal Number		
Palmer's Notation		
Eruption Date		
Antagonists		
Succedaneous		
Number of Cusps		
Number of Roots		
*Identifying Features**		
Buccal		
Lingual		
Mesial		
Distal		
Occlusal Description		
Cusps		
Fossae		
Grooves		

*Size, number of cusps, location of grooves, etc.

CHAPTER 11

Mandibular First and Second Molars

General Information
Mandibular First Molar
Mandibular Second Molar

OBJECTIVES

- Identify the mandibular first and second molars and provide vital information: that is, universal number, function, antagonist, and so forth.
- Describe the location and contour of each first and second molar.
- Define the new terms in the chapter.
- Complete the worksheet at the end of the chapter.

GENERAL INFORMATION

There are six mandibular molars: three in each quadrant. As with the maxillary molars, they are named for their position in the arch: first, second, and third molar. Again, molars erupt posterior to the primary second molars and are not succedaneous teeth.

The mandibular first molar is the first permanent tooth to erupt, and its positioning in the arch is important for the appropriate **alignment** of the other permanent teeth. (See Chapter 15, "Occlusion.") Therefore, it is considered the "**keystone**" of the dental arch.

Mandibular molars have either four or five cusps; the number of lobes from which they develop is the same as the number of cusps. The roots of mandibular molars are **bifurcated** (divided in two) into a mesial and distal root. Although each root of a tooth usually has one pulp canal, the mandibular first molar is the exception and has two pulp canals in the mesial root. The major function of the mandibular molars is to assist the maxillary molars with grinding and pulverizing the food.

MANDIBULAR FIRST MOLAR

Characteristics

Location in the Arch . . . . Sixth tooth from the midline; distal to second premolar

Universal Number . . . . R-#30   L-#19

Eruption Date . . . . 6–7 years

First Evidence of Calcification . . . . . Birth

Crown Completion . . . . $2^1/_2$–3 years

Root Completion . . . . 9–10 years

Function . . . . Mastication and comminution of food

Length of Crown . . . . 7.5 mm

Length of Root . . . . 14 mm

Antagonists . . . . Maxillary second premolar and first molar

Location of Contact Area

Mesial . . . . Occlusal third

Distal . . . . Occlusal third

Identifying Features

- five cusps: mesiobuccal, distobuccal, distal, mesiolingual, distolingual
- two roots: mesial and distal
- three pulp canals: two in mesial root, one in distal root
- largest mandibular tooth
- first permanent tooth to erupt

(Refer to Figure 11-1)

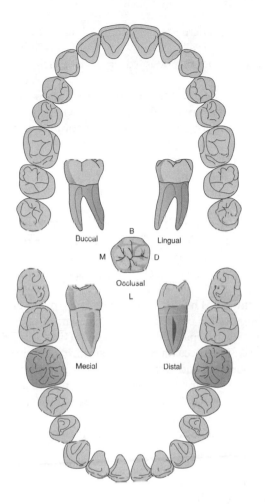

FIGURE 11-1
Mandibular first molars

Tooth Description of the Mandibular First Molar

Buccal Surface.   Three buccal cusps and the tips of the two higher lingual cusps can be seen. The buccal cusps are flat and separated by grooves (Figure 11-2). The cusps, in order of size, are mesiobuccal, distobuccal, and distal. They are divided by the mesiobuccal and distobuccal grooves, respectively. Slight depressions are at the base of each groove.

The *mesial side*, from cervix to contact area, is concave, becoming convex at the contact area in the occlusal third. The *distal side* is straight from cervix to contact area, where it becomes convex. The contact area is located slightly more toward the occlusal than on the mesial side.

The cervical line curves slightly in an apical direction. The root trunk, about 3 mm in length, bifurcates into a mesial and distal root. For half its length, the mesial root curves mesially; then it curves toward the distal. The distal root is less curved and slants in a distal direction.

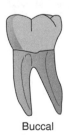

Buccal

FIGURE 11-2
Mandibular first molar—
buccal surface

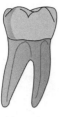

Lingual

FIGURE 11-3
Mandibular first molar—
lingual surface

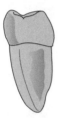

Mesial

FIGURE 11-4
Mandibular first molar—
mesial surface

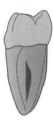

Distal

FIGURE 11-5
Mandibular first molar—distal
surface

Lingual Surface.   There are two pointed lingual cusps, the mesiolingual and distolingual, divided by a lingual groove (Figure 11-3). The **distal cusp** can also be seen. At the root bifurcation is a deep developmental groove.

Mesial Surface.   Because the tooth is broader on the mesial side, only the mesiobuccal and mesiolingual cusps are seen (Figure 11-4). They are joined by the mesial marginal ridge, located about 1 mm below the cusp tips. The cervical line curves 1 mm in an occlusal direction.

Extending from the contact area and continuing onto the root is a shallow depression. The root remains broad for almost its entire length, tapering only at the apical third. This mesial root usually has two pulp canals.

Distal Surface.   Because the crown converges toward the distal, a portion of the buccal surface is seen. The distal portion of the crown is also shorter, such that all the cusps are visible (Figure 11-5). A relatively straight cervical line separates the crown and the root. A shallow depression is present on the distal root.

Occlusal Surface.   The dimensions are wider from mesial to distal than from buccal to lingual, the opposite of the maxillary molar. All five cusps are functioning cusps, each separated by a groove (Figure 11-6). The occlusal grooves extend from the buccal and lingual surface and have the same names: mesiobuccal, distobuccal, and lingual. These three grooves form a Y-shape. They each join the central groove, which goes from mesial to distal across the center of the occlusal surface. There is a deep **central pit** where grooves merge.

The sides of each cusp slope to form fossae. There is a large central circular fossa as well as mesial and distal triangular fossae.

CLINICAL CONSIDERATIONS
Root length: 14 mm
Root depressions: (1) On the buccal surface, a deep depression extending into the root bifurcation 3 mm from the cervical line; (2) on the lingual surface, a deep developmental depression at bifurcation; (3) on the mesial surface, a broad but shallow depression extending from the crown down the root surface; and (4) on the distal surface, a shallow depression extending most of root length.
CEJ: Very slight curvature (0–1 mm toward occlusal) on both mesial and distal surfaces.
Cervical area from buccal or lingual surface: Mesial side is concave; distal surface is straight.
Furcation: Buccal surface is 3 mm from cervical line; lingual surface is 3–4 mm from the cervical line.

Summary of the Mandibular First Molar

Buccal Surface.   The characteristics of this surface are:

Crown

• Three flat buccal cusps: mesiobuccal, distobuccal, and distal.

Grooves

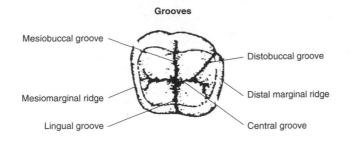

Mesiobuccal groove

Distobuccal groove

Mesiomarginal ridge

Distal marginal ridge

Lingual groove

Central groove

Fossae

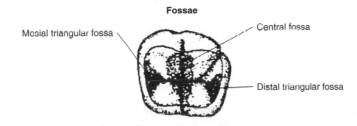

Mesial triangular fossa

Central fossa

Distal triangular fossa

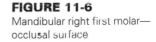

FIGURE 11-6
Mandibular right first molar—occlusal surface

- Five cusps are visible as the lingual cusps are longer and more pointed.
- Mesiobuccal and distobuccal grooves divide the cusps.
- Slight depression or pit at the base of each groove.
- A concave mesial side.
- A mesial contact area in the occlusal third.
- A straight distal side.
- A distal contact area that is more occlusal than the mesial contact area.

Root

- The mesial root curves mesially for half its length, then curves distally.
- The distal root is less curved, with its axis in a distal direction.
- The root bifurcates about 3 mm below the cervical line and has a deep developmental depression.

Lingual Surface.   The characteristics of this surface are:

Crown

- Two pointed lingual cusps: mesiolingual and distolingual.
- A visible distal cusp.
- The lingual groove divides the lingual cusps.

Roots
- A deep developmental depression at the root bifurcation.

Mesial Surface.   The characteristics of this surface are:

Crown

- Two visible cusps: mesiobuccal and mesiolingual.
- Mesial marginal ridge located about 1 mm below cusp tips.

- Cervical line curves occlusally about 1 mm.
- Concave area at the cervical line that continues onto the root.

Root

- Only the mesial root is visible.
- Mesial root usually has two pulp canals.
- Broad and straight root, tapering in the apical third.
- A broad concavity or depression on the root.

Distal Surface.   The characteristics of this surface are:

Crown

- Tooth converges toward distal so that some of the buccal surface is seen.
- Crown is shorter on the distal so that all cusps are seen.
- Relatively straight cervical line.

Root

- A shallow depression is often evident on the root.

Occlusal Surface.   The characteristics of this surface are:
- Dimensions are wider (by 1 mm) from distal to mesial than from buccal to lingual.
- Five functioning cusps, in order of size, are mesiolingual, mesiobuccal, distolingual, distobuccal, and distal.
- Major grooves: central, mesiobuccal, distobuccal, and lingual (Y-shape).
- Major fossae: central (circular), mesial, and distal triangular (Figure 11-6).
- Pits: central, mesial, and distal.

MANDIBULAR SECOND MOLAR

Characteristics

Location in the Arch	Seventh tooth from the midline; distal to the first molar
Universal Number.	R-#31 L-#18
Eruption Date.	11–13 years
First Evidence of Calcification	$2\frac{1}{2}$–3 years
Crown Completion	7–8 years
Root Completion	14–15 years
Function	Mastication and comminution
Length of Crown	7 mm
Length of Root.	13 mm
Antagonists	Maxillary first and second molars

Location of Contact Area

Mesial	Occlusal third
Distal	Occlusal third

(continues)

MANDIBULAR SECOND MOLAR (continued)

Identifying Features
- four cusps: mesiobuccal, distobuccal, mesiolingual, distolingual
- two roots: mesial and distal
- two pulp canals: one in each root

(Refer to Figure 11-7)

Tooth Description of the Mandibular Second Molar

Because of its similarity to the first molar, only the structural variations of the mandibular second molar are listed below (see Figure 11-8).

- It is smaller.
- There are only four cusps: mesiobuccal, distobuccal, mesiolingual, distolingual.
- The buccal groove divides the two buccal cusps and continues onto the occlusal surface.

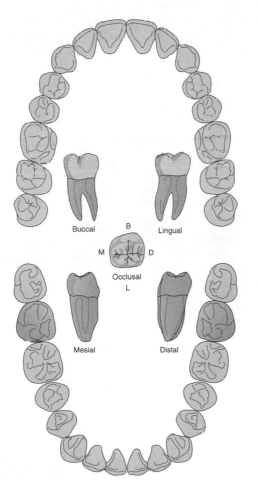

FIGURE 11-7
Mandibular second molars

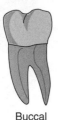
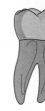

Buccal   Lingual

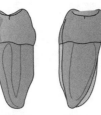

Mesial   Distal

FIGURE 11-8

Mandibular second molar — buccal, lingual, mesial, and distal surfaces

- The lingual groove divides the two lingual cusps and continues onto the occlusal surface.
- The mesial side of the tooth is wider (from buccal to lingual) than the distal. Therefore the mesial cusps are larger than the distal cusps.
- The occlusal groove pattern, shown in Figure 11-9:

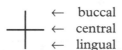

- ← buccal
- ← central
- ← lingual

- The occlusal has more supplementary grooves.
- The mesial root has only one pulp canal.

CLINICAL CONSIDERATIONS

Root length: 13 mm

Root depressions: (1) On buccal surface, the root bifurcation is 3 mm from cervical line; (2) on lingual surface, a deep developmental groove is evident at the bifurcation; (3) on mesial surface, a shallow depression extends from crown down the root surface; and (4) on distal surface, a shallow depression extends most of root length.

CEJ: Very slight curvature (0–1 mm toward occlusal) on both mesial and distal surfaces.

Cervical area from buccal or lingual surface: The mesial side is concave; the distal surface is straight.

Furcation: Buccal surface is 3 mm from cervical line; lingual surface is 3–4 mm from cervical line.

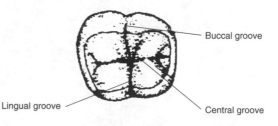

Buccal groove

Lingual groove

Central groove

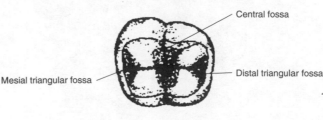

Central fossa

Distal triangular fossa

Mesial triangular fossa

FIGURE 11-9

Mandibular second molar— occlusal surface

SUMMARY

Each mandibular quadrant has three mandibular molars. The mandibular first molar is usually the first permanent tooth to erupt, so its positioning is important for the appropriate alignment of the other permanent teeth. Thus, it is the "keystone" to the arch.

The mandibular first molar has five cusps, three buccal and two lingual; the second molar has four cusps, two buccal and two lingual.

Mandibular molars have two roots, one mesial and one distal. All teeth have one pulp canal in each root, but the mandibular first molar is often the exception. There are three pulp canals in the two roots: the mesial root has two pulp canals, the distal root has one pulp canal. The mandibular second molar has only one pulp canal in each root.

The mandibular molars assist the maxillary molars in **mastication** and comminution.

WORKSHEET

A. Complete the following chart with the information requested.

	Mandibular First Molar	Mandibular Second Molar
Universal Number		
Palmer's Notation		
Eruption Date		
Antagonists		
Succedaneous		
Number of Cusps		
Number of Roots		
Identifying Features*		
Buccal		
Lingual		
Mesial		
Distal		
Occlusal Description		
Cusps		
Fossae		
Grooves		

*Size, number of cusps, location of grooves, etc.

Third Molars

General Information
Maxillary Third Molar
Mandibular Third Molar

OBJECTIVES

- Identify the third molars and provide vital information: that is, universal number, function, antagonist, and so forth.
- Describe the location and contour of each third molar.
- Define the new terms in the chapter.
- Complete the worksheet at the end of the chapter.
- Perform the clinical applications at the end of the chapter.

GENERAL INFORMATION

Because both maxillary and mandibular third molars show considerable developmental variation, there is no standard structural description. These teeth, more than any of the others, are likely to be **anomalies**. Often, there is crown displacement and the roots are fused or malformed.

When the third molars develop properly, their structure will look like either the first or second molar, but they can be differentiated because they are smaller and will have numerous supplementary grooves on the occlusal surface. The root will usually be fused even when the crown is not malformed.

Third molars supplement the other molars in grinding food. Although it is not necessary to study the structure of third molars, it is helpful to examine specimens to realize their difference from other molars.

MAXILLARY THIRD MOLAR

Characteristics
Location in the Arch . . . . Eighth tooth from midline; distal to maxillary second molar
Universal Number . . . . R-#1   L-#16
Eruption Date . . . . 17–21 years
First Evidence of Calcification . . . . . 7–9 years
Crown Completion . . . . 12–16 years
Root Completion . . . . 18–25 years
Function . . . . Mastication and comminution
Length of Crown . . . . 6.5 mm
Length of Root . . . . 11 mm
Antagonists . . . . Mandibular third molar

Location of Contact Area
Mesial . . . . variation from middle to
Distal . . . . occlusal third

Identifying Features
- often the crown is heart-shaped
- fused roots (three roots)
- may resemble first or second molar

(Refer to Figure 12-1)

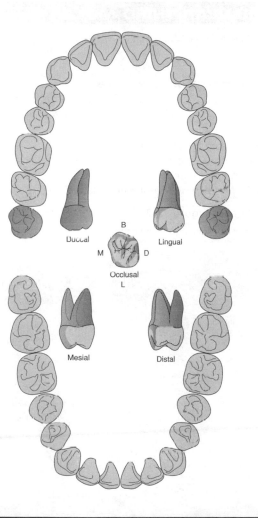

FIGURE 12-1
Maxillary third molars

MANDIBULAR THIRD MOLAR

Characteristics

Location in the Arch	Eighth tooth from midline; distal to mandibular second molar
Universal Number	R-#32 L-#17
Eruption Date	17–21 years
First Evidence of Calcification	8–10 years
Crown Completion	12–16 years
Root Completion	18–25 years
Function	Mastication and comminution
Length of Crown	7 mm
Length of Root	11 mm

(continues)

MANDIBULAR THIRD MOLAR (continued)

Antagonists . . . . Maxillary second and third molars

Location of Contact Area

Mesial . . . . variation from middle to
Distal . . . . occlusal third

Identifying Features

- often crowns do not conform to normal size
- often have fused roots
- when well developed will look like first or second molar

(Refer to Figure 12-2)

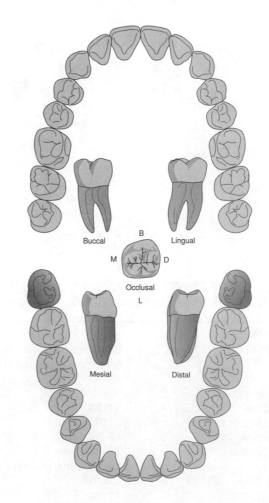

FIGURE 12-2
Mandibular third molars

SUMMARY

Because of developmental variations, there is no standard description for the maxillary or mandibular third molars. When well formed, they will be smaller than but similar to the first molars in number of cusps and roots. Usually, however, the roots are fused and the crowns will have numerous **supplemental** (small, indistinct) **grooves**. Frequently, the maxillary third molar is **heart-shaped**, but the mandibular third molar is often atypical.

WORKSHEET

Answer the following questions as completely as possible:

1. What is the most common shape of the crown of the maxillary third molar?

2. What is a common feature of the roots of both maxillary and mandibular third molars?

3. What maxillary and mandibular third molars develop normally, what do they resemble?

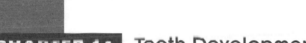

Related Topics

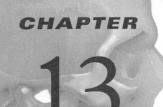

Primary Dentition

KEY TERMS

Deciduous

Primate spacing

Eruption

Exfoliation

Mixed dentition

Cervical ridge

Flared (divergent) roots

OBJECTIVES

- Identify the names, number, and eruption dates of the primary teeth.
- Describe the value of the primary teeth to function.
- Compare the primary teeth to the permanent teeth.
- Complete the worksheet at the end of the chapter.
- Perform the clinical applications at the end of the chapter.

THE NAMES AND NUMBER OF THE PRIMARY TEETH

There are twenty primary teeth: ten maxillary and ten mandibular. In each quadrant there is a central incisor, lateral incisor, canine, first molar, and second molar (Figure 13-1). There are no premolars in the primary dentition. Primary teeth are also referred to as **deciduous** teeth, baby teeth, milk teeth, or first teeth.

ERUPTION/EXFOLIATION

The period of eruption for the primary teeth occurs from 6 months to $2^1/_2$–3 years of age. The specific eruption date for each tooth is listed in Appendix A. All the primary teeth usually have emerged and are in alignment by the time the child is 3 years old. Although each permanent tooth contacts its proximal tooth, there is spacing between each anterior primary tooth. This spacing, called **primate spacing**, allows for the development and growth of the larger succedaneous tooth forming in the bone beneath each primary tooth. Primate spaces are usually located between the primary maxillary lateral incisor and canine, and between the primary mandibular canine and first molar.

At 6 years, just prior to the **eruption** of the permanent mandibular central incisor, exfoliation of the primary teeth begins. The mandibular central incisors are the first to exfoliate. The **exfoliation** sequence is the same as the eruption sequence of the permanent dentition.

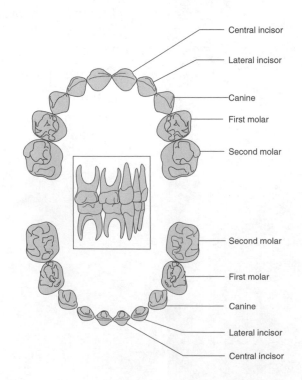

Central incisor

Lateral incisor

Canine

First molar

Second molar

Second molar

First molar

Canine

Lateral incisor

Central incisor

FIGURE 13-1

The primary dentition with tooth identification

During the period when both deciduous and permanent teeth are present in the oral cavity, the person has a **mixed dentition**. By about 12 years of age, all primary teeth are normally replaced by permanent teeth.

COMPARISON WITH PERMANENT TEETH

All primary anterior teeth resemble their permanent counterparts although they are smaller (Figure 13-2). The primary first molars have several cusps, and although they can be identified as molars, they are not anatomically identical to any permanent tooth. All primary second molars resemble the first permanent molars.

Primary teeth have a more pronounced **cervical ridge**. In addition, the **roots** of the posterior teeth are more **flared (divergent)**, thus allowing for growth of the permanent teeth forming beneath them. Because the roots are flared, the cervix appears to be more constricted than the cervix of the permanent teeth.

The primary crowns have less enamel than do the permanent teeth, and the pulp horns extend more occlusally than on the permanent teeth. Therefore, the pulp is closer to the surface. Special consideration must be given to reducing excessive friction when rubber cup polishing these teeth since the heat could cause injury to the pulp.

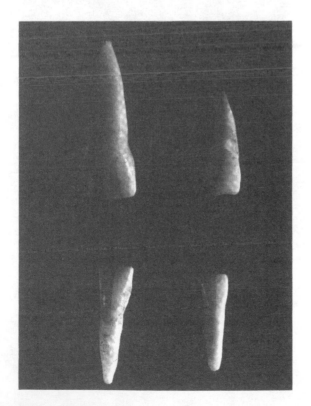

FIGURE 13-2
Primary incisors compared to permanent incisors

Once you have become familiar with permanent tooth anatomy, you can more easily differentiate the primary teeth from permanent teeth in the clinical examination.

DESCRIPTION OF PRIMARY TEETH

Maxillary Teeth

Incisors.   The labial crown of the incisor is smooth with a straight incisal edge; there are no mamelons. The crown is wide with a cingulum and marginal ridges on the lingual.

Canine.   A broad cervical ridge on the canine causes the cervix to appear constricted. The cusp tip is pointed, but short; the root is long and slender (Figure 13-3).

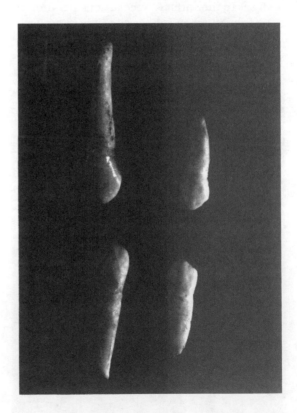

FIGURE 13-3

Primary canines compared to permanent canines

First Molar.   The number of cusps varies from 2 to 4. There is no groove on the buccal surface to divide the cusps.

The occlusal surface has a central fossa and a mesial triangular fossa connected by a central groove. There are three roots on all maxillary molars, and the bifurcation of the two buccal roots begins almost apically to the cervix.

Second Molar.   The anatomy is the same as that of the permanent maxillary first molar (Figure 13-4). There are two buccal cusps divided by a buccal groove and two lingual cusps with a cusp of Carabelli, or fifth cusp groove, on the mesiolingual cusp. There are three roots: two buccal, one lingual.

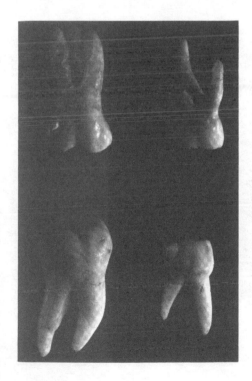

FIGURE 13-4
Primary molars compared to permanent molars

Mandibular Teeth

Incisors.   Both labial and lingual surfaces are smooth, although there is a slight cingulum and marginal ridges on the lingual.

Canines.   The buccal surface has a pronounced cervical ridge. The lingual surface has a cingulum and lingual ridges.

First Molar.   As with the maxillary first molar, there is no definite anatomy. Usually there are two buccal cusps divided by a depression, rather than a groove, and two lingual cusps. There are two roots; both are long, slender, and divergent. The occlusal surface has a central groove crossed by the buccal groove and a lingual groove.

Second Molar.   The anatomy is identical to that of the permanent mandibular first molar. Grooves divide the three buccal cusps and the two lingual cusps. The occlusal groove pattern is also the same as that on the permanent mandibular first molar, although there may be more supplemental grooves. There are two long, thin, divergent roots, which can be twice as long as the crown.

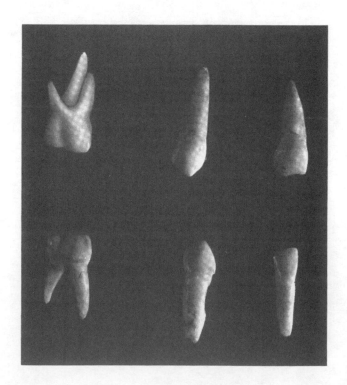

FIGURE 13-5

Primary incisors, canines, and molars

IMPORTANCE OF PRIMARY TEETH

Both the form and function of the primary dentition are important (Figure 13-5). Each primary tooth has the same function as the permanent tooth that succeeds it, and each maintains a position for its permanent tooth replacement. If prematurely lost, the permanent replacement may erupt too early or emerge in an incorrect position. This may result in improper alignment and cause future malocclusion and periodontal problems. Because of these factors, it is important to stress care and maintenance of the primary teeth with the patient. The deciduous molars must be in a condition to function for 10–12 years. The development of good dental habits during these early years will result in a healthier permanent dentition.

SUMMARY

The primary dentition includes 10 maxillary and 10 mandibular teeth. Eruption begins around the 6th month of life and is completed between $2^1/_2$ and 3 years. Each primary tooth resembles its succeeding permanent tooth but is proportionately smaller. The posterior teeth have flared roots that allow for concurrent growth of the permanent teeth growing directly below.

The primary teeth are an important part of the dentition; each of these teeth has a necessary function. It is important that they are cared for so that they endure until their natural exfoliation.

WORKSHEET

A. Review the eruption sequence of the deciduous teeth. List the teeth in the correct sequence of eruption.

_____

_____

_____

_____

_____

_____

_____

_____

_____

_____

Tooth Development

Introduction
Growth and Development
Eruption
Developmental Anomalies

OBJECTIVES

- Describe the development of the tooth during the following stages: growth (initiation, proliferation, histodifferentiation, and morphodifferentiation), apposition, and calcification.
- Define: active and passive eruption, proliferation, histodifferentiation, morphodifferentiation, apposition, supernumerary, and anomaly.
- Complete the worksheet at the end of the chapter.

INTRODUCTION

The development of a human begins with an embryo, which has three layers: the **ectoderm**, the **mesoderm**, and the **endoderm**. The ectoderm will form not only the outer covering of the body but also the lining of the oral cavity. The skeletal and muscular systems, as well as other structures including the cementum, dentin, and pulp of the tooth, form from the mesoderm. The lining of the internal organs develops from the endoderm.

During the third week of fetal life, when the embryo is only 3 mm long, the face begins its development. At one end of the embryo there is an invagination of the ectoderm forming the **stomodeum**, or primitive mouth, which later becomes the oral and nasal cavities.

The primitive mouth is lined with ectoderm and becomes the oral epithelium. Beneath this is the mesenchyme, developed from mesoderm, which becomes the underlying connective tissue.

Between the fifth and sixth week in utero, the first sign of tooth development is evident. Teeth are formed from the ectoderm and mesoderm in a complex histologic process simplified into the following pattern.

GROWTH AND DEVELOPMENT

The following information is taken from Phinney and Halstead, *Dental Assisting*, 89–90 (Thomson Delmar Learning, 2000).

The growth stage is defined by an increase in the number and size of the cells (Figure 14-1). The formation of the teeth is a progression that begins during the fifth or sixth week in utero with the formation of the primary mandibular anterior teeth, followed shortly by the development of the primary maxillary anterior teeth. This developmental process continues, posteriorly, until 10 maxillary and 10 mandibular teeth are formed. Permanent teeth begin forming about the fourth or fifth month of fetal life but do not calcify until after birth.

Initiation—Bud Stage

The first stage of *odontogenesis* (origin of the tooth) is referred to as the *bud stage*. During this stage, initiation takes place. **Initiation** is when the tooth begins formation from the *dental lamina*. The dental lamina is a growth from the oral epithelium that gives rise to the tooth buds. Therefore, on a deciduous dentition, ten growths on each arch are apparent or ten buds later become the primary teeth. The first sign of a developing tooth is noted during the embryonic phase in the area that will eventually be the lower mandibular anterior region of the child's oral cavity. The permanent teeth develop in a similar manner. Each arch has sixteen different buds developing into one tooth each. The last three molars in each quadrant develop behind the primary dentition. The six-year molar begins developing at birth, the twelve-year molar starts developing when the baby is about six months old, and the third molars (wisdom teeth) start when the child is approximately five years of age.

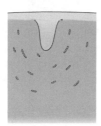

(A) Initiation

Bud stage

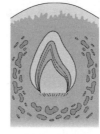

(E) Apposition

Maturation stage

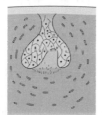

(B) Proliferation

Cap stage (begins proliferation,
histodifferentiation,
and morphodifferentiation

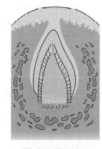

(F) Calcification

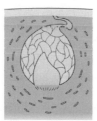

(C) Histodifferentiation

Bell stage

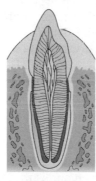

(G) Eruption

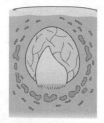

(D) Morphodifferentiation

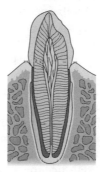

(H) Attrition

FIGURE 14-1

Stages of tooth development

Proliferation—Cap Stage

The bud of the tooth grows and changes shape during the cap stage. The organ is indented on the lower side and appears much like a cap, therefore the name *cap stage*. The primary embryonic ectoderm layer that has developed into the oral epithelium matures into the enamel of the developing tooth. The processes of **proliferation**, when the cells multiply, and **histodifferentiation**, when the cells develop into different tissues, take place along with early **morphodifferentiation**, when the cells begin to outline the future shape of the developing organ. During this process, the primary embryonic mesoderm layer develops into connective tissue that is referred to as the *mesenchyme* tissue. This connective tissue forms an enclosed area, referred to as a *dental sac*, and further matures into the dentin, cementum, and the pulp of the tooth. A portion of the mesenchyme surrounds the outside of the enamel organ, the cementum, and the periodontal ligament of the tooth.

Morphodifferentiation/Histodifferentiation— Bell Stage

Further specialization of the cells, or histodifferentiation, takes place in the bell stage. The inner epithelium of the enamel organ becomes *ameloblasts*, enamel-forming cells. The peripheral cells of the dental papilla become *odontoblasts*, cells that form dentin. The *cementoblasts*, cementum-forming cells, form from the dental sac. Continued morphodifferentiation takes place, forming the organ into a shape that resembles a bell.

Apposition—Maturation State

The odontogenesis reaches completion in these final stages. The tissues of enamel, dentin, and cementum are formed in layers and fused together in the appropriate manner. The process of depositing calcium salts and other minerals in the formed tooth takes place during the **apposition** stage. This process is called **calcification** and is the last developmental state prior to *eruption* of the tooth. The final stage of the life cycle of the tooth is *attrition*, or the wearing away of the incisal or occlusal surfaces of the tooth during normal function.

The root of the tooth does not develop fully prior to eruption. Eruption is the phase when the tooth passes through the bone and the oral mucosa and into its place in the oral cavity. Twenty of the permanent teeth are located below and distal to the primary teeth. As the permanent teeth erupt, they apply pressure to the apices of the roots of the primary teeth. During this force, *osteoclasts*, bone resorption cells, dissolve the root of the primary tooth. This resorption first takes place at the apex and continues up toward the crown of the tooth. When very little of the root structure of the primary tooth is left, the tooth loosens because of lack of support. Children often assist in the final stages of loosening the tooth by moving it back and forth until they break the attaching fibers.

The primary teeth occupy and maintain space in the dental arches for the permanent teeth and act as guides during the eruption process. If the primary teeth are removed early, the spaces may be diminished, causing crowding when the permanent teeth erupt.

ERUPTION

Eruption is the movement of the tooth from its position within the jaw to its position in the oral cavity. The process is divided into active and passive eruption.

Active Eruption

This is the process whereby the crown of the tooth first moves from within the jaw into the oral cavity, a process that continues until the tooth meets its antagonist in the opposite jaw. **Active eruption** begins when the crown of the tooth is complete and a portion of the root has started to form. When the tooth emerges into the oral cavity, only a portion of the root has formed, as previously described.

It will take $1^1/_2$ to 3 years for the completion of a deciduous root and about 3 years after eruption for the completion of a permanent root. The entire process of permanent tooth development, from initiation to completion, takes about 10 years.

By the time a primary tooth erupts, its succedaneous replacement, the permanent tooth, has begun forming. With the exception of the permanent molars, this occurs beneath the root(s) of the deciduous tooth. Again, refer to the chart on tooth development in Chapter 1 for a review of the growth rate of teeth. Note that the first permanent molars begin calcifying after birth and develop in the area posterior to the second deciduous molars.

Passive Eruption

Once active eruption is complete, other factors that occur during life, such as wear from use or trauma, can cause attrition or breakdown on the periodontium. In turn, there can be exposure of cementum, wearing of the enamel, or gingival recession. The increase in the length of the clinical crown caused by gingival recession is referred to as **passive eruption**.

DEVELOPMENTAL ANOMALIES

Disturbances in the development stage of the teeth and bones can cause abnormalities. Hereditary or nutritional factors, such as excessive amounts of fluoride, may cause an **anomaly**, or deviation in the development of the teeth.

For example, any disturbance or interference in the fusion of the right and left maxillary process can result in a cleft of the palate. Disturbances during the formation of the tooth structure can cause faulty enamel or alteration of the shape of the tooth. Examples of this are enamel dysphasia, fluorosis, or peg-shaped lateral incisors. Occasionally, there may be an extra tooth that has formed called a **supernumerary** tooth. It is helpful to review oral-histology literature detailing the explanation of the causes of various tooth abnormalities in order to more clearly understand when and how these deviations occur.

SUMMARY

Between the fifth and sixth week in utero, there is evidence of tooth development. An increase in growth and development of the cells continues until the entire tooth is formed, a process that lasts 2–3 years for the primary teeth and 9–10 years for the permanent teeth. Once a tooth is formed, it cannot repair itself as bones and skin do. It is necessary to provide a proper diet during tooth formation and preventive care after eruption so that the teeth will last a lifetime.

WORKSHEET

A. *Number each stage of development in the order it occurs, and describe what occurs at each stage.*

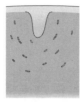 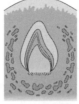

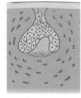 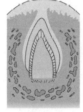

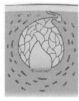 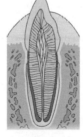

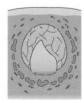 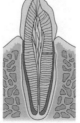

Occlusion

Occlusion
Ideal Occlusion
Normal Occlusion
Malocclusion
Occlusal Deviations
Angle's Classification of Occlusion
Related Terms
Primary Teeth Occlusion

OBJECTIVES

- Describe Angle's classification of occlusion.
- Describe five occlusal deviations that affect a group of teeth, and explain the importance of primary teeth spacing on the occlusion of permanent teeth.
- List and explain five deviations of individual tooth positioning.
- Describe three types of facial profiles.
- Define the following terms: ideal occlusion, normal occlusion, malocclusion, centric occlusion, centric relation, terminal mesial step, terminal plane, and primate spacing.
- Complete the worksheet at the end of the chapter.
- Perform the clinical applications at the end of the chapter.

OCCLUSION

Occlusion occurs when the maxillary and mandibular teeth contact each other in any functional relationship. The study of occlusion is concerned with all the factors involved in the development, stability, and function of the **masticatory** system, not only with the contacting of the teeth. The masticatory system includes the teeth and surrounding structures, jaws, temporomandibular joint (TMJ), muscles, lips, tongue, and related nerves and blood vessels. Thus, the study of occlusion can be complex, extending beyond the arrangement of the teeth to include areas such as growth and development of the entire masticatory system—that is, genetic as well as environmental factors.

Occlusion first occurs after the eruption of the primary dentition. The sequence of eruption, spacing, and positioning of the teeth as well as the relationship of the jaws can be critical to occlusion, particularly if they vary significantly from the normal. The final occlusal relationship of the permanent dentition is a result of the influence of hereditary and environmental factors such as trauma, oral habits, or faulty dental treatment.

IDEAL OCCLUSION

Ideal occlusion implies a complete, harmonious relationship of the teeth, as well as of all other structures involved in the masticatory system (Figure 15-1). In an ideal anatomic occlusal relationship, as S. Ramfjord and M. Ash have noted, the teeth conform to a specific pattern that includes 138 occlusal contacts in the closure of the 32 permanent teeth. This ideal relationship, however, rarely exists.

When the maxillary and mandibular teeth are in an ideal position, the maxillary teeth facially overlap the mandibular teeth by one-third, and each maxillary tooth has a distal relationship to its mandibular counterpart by the distance of about one-half a tooth. Lingual cusps of maxillary posterior teeth occlude in specific fossae of mandibular teeth. An intercusp relationship such as this is referred to as interdigitation.

Ideal occlusion is noted, also, by the positioning of the permanent first molars and canines. The mesiobuccal cusp of the maxillary first molar will be positioned in the mesiobuccal groove of the mandibular first molar. And

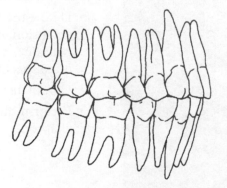

FIGURE 15-1
Permanent teeth in occlusion

the maxillary canine will occlude in the middle of the mandibular canine and the mandibular first premolar.

NORMAL OCCLUSION

As ideal occlusion seldom occurs, **normal occlusion** conforms closely to an ideal occlusal relationship but involves some variations from it. With normal occlusion, variations are considered optimum if there is functional comfort and stability of alignment. Normal or optimum occlusion is needed to maintain or protect the periodontium and/or TMJ, as well as for stabilization of alignment and aesthetics.

It is necessary that each tooth be able to withstand the forces exerted during mastication. The biting force of the posterior teeth is about 100–170 pounds. According to Ralph W. Phillips in *Elements of Dental Materials*, this represents 28,000 pounds per square inch or 300 pounds of pressure exerted by pressing down on a point with a medium-sharp pencil. In proper occlusion, each tooth has an appropriate opposing contact. A malpositioned tooth can cause improper distribution of stress, resulting in a breakdown of the periodontium and/or TMJ pathology.

According to Dr. Edward Angle, in a normal relationship, the first permanent molars are considered the key to occlusion and their position is the same as an ideal occlusion: the mesiobuccal cusp of the maxillary first molar rests in the mesiobuccal groove of the mandibular first molar.

MALOCCLUSION

Any deviation from ideal positioning of the teeth, whether it is a minor deviation of one tooth or a severe variation involving several teeth or the jaws, creates a **malocclusion**. The best-known system for classifying malocclusions was first described by Dr. Angle in 1898. His system is based on the mesiodistal relationship of the maxillary and mandibular first molars and canines to each other—the maxillary first molar being his "key" to occlusion. Any variation in this relationship constitutes a malocclusion.

OCCLUSAL DEVIATIONS

Malocclusion or malalignment can affect an individual tooth or several teeth (refer to Table 15-1). Occlusal deviations involving several teeth are:

- **Openbite**—an existing space between the mandibular and maxillary teeth. An openbite can be
  a. anterior or
  b. posterior—unilateral or bilateral.
- **Overbite**—a deep or vertical overlap of the maxillary teeth onto the mandibular teeth that exceeds the normal, or one-third the depth of the mandibular incisors.

- **Overjet**—a horizontal overlap creating a protrusion or space between the labial surface of the mandibular incisors and the lingual surface of the maxillary incisors.
- **Crossbite**—a facially positioned mandibular tooth, or teeth. This can be
  a. anterior or
  b. posterior—buccal or lingual.

TABLE 15-1   MALPOSITIONS OF GROUPS OF TEETH

Term	Description	Illustration
Anterior crossbite	Abnormal relationship of a tooth or a group of teeth in one arch to the opposing teeth in the other arch. In anterior crossbite the maxillary incisors are positioned lingually to the opposing mandibular incisors.	
Posterior crossbite	Abnormal relationship of teeth in one arch to the opposing teeth in the other arch. In posterior crossbite the primary or permanent maxillary posterior teeth are positioned lingually to the mandibular teeth.	
Edge-to-edge bite	Incisal surfaces of maxillary anterior teeth meeting the incisal surfaces of mandibular anterior teeth.	
End-to-end bite	Maxillary posterior teeth meeting mandibular posterior teeth cusp-to-cusp instead of in the normal fashion.	
Openbite	Failure of the maxillary and mandibular to occlude (meet).	

TABLE 15-1   MALPOSITIONS OF GROUPS OF TEETH (continued)

Term	Description	Illustration
Overjet (horizontal overlap)	An abnormal horizontal distance between the labial surface of mandibular anterior teeth and the labial surface of maxillary anterior teeth.	
Overbite (vertical overlap)	Normally the maxillary teeth extend vertically over the incisal one-third of the mandibular anterior teeth. When the vertical overlap is greater than this, the person is said to have an overbite.	
Underjet	Maxillary anteriors positioned lingually to mandibular anteriors with excessive space between labial of maxillary anteriors and lingual of mandibular anteriors.	

- **Edge-to-edge** or **end-to-end**—a contacting of the incisal edges or cusp tips rather than an interdigitation of cusp and fossae. Actually, this is a crossbite or precrossbite condition.
- **Underjet**—a horizontal relationship where the maxillary anteriors are lingual to the mandibular anteriors.

Occlusal deviations involving individual teeth are:

- **Labioversion** or **buccoversion**—a tooth positioned more facially than normal (Figure 15-2).
- **Linguoversion**—a tooth positioned more lingually than normal (Figure 15-3).
- **Infraversion**—a tooth positioned below the plane of occlusion (Figure 15-4).
- **Supraversion**—a tooth positioned above the plane of occlusion (Figure 15-5).
- **Torsoversion**—a rotated tooth (Figure 15-6).

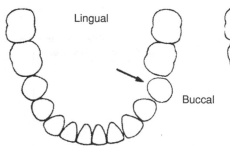

FIGURE 15-2
Buccoversion

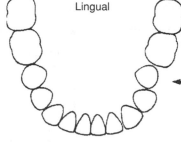

FIGURE 15-3
Linguoversion

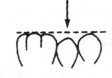

FIGURE 15-4
Infraversion

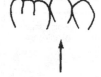

FIGURE 15-5
Supraversion

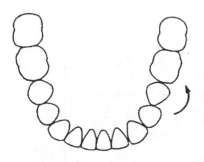

FIGURE 15-6
Torsoversion

ANGLE'S CLASSIFICATION OF OCCLUSION

Dr. Angle was the first to develop a system to classify malocclusion. Because the mandible is movable, **Angle's classification** relates to the anterior–posterior or mesiodistal deviations in relation to the first molar. There are three classifications (see Table 15-2).

Class I—Neutrocclusion (Normal)

Both the permanent first molar and canine relationship are in ideal position. The mesiobuccal cusp of the maxillary first molar rests in the mesiobuccal groove of the mandibular first molar, and the maxillary canine occludes with the distal inclined plane of the mandibular canine and the mandibular first premolar.

In a Class I relationship there can be deviations of a single tooth or several anterior teeth such as an overjet or overbite, but the molars will have ideal positioning.

TABLE 15-2 ANGLE'S CLASSIFICATIONS OF MALOCCLUSION AND FACIAL PROFILES

Class name	Molar relationship	Description	Illustration	Facial profile
Neutrocclusion	Mesiobuccal cusp of maxillary first permanent molar occludes with the buccal groove of mandibular first permanent molar.	Similar to normal occlusion with individual teeth or groups of teeth out of position.	Class I	Mesognathic
Distocclusion	Buccal groove of the mandibular first permanent molar is distal to mesiobuccal cusp of maxillary first permanent molar.	Division 1— maxillary teeth in labioversion.	Class II, Division 1	Retrognathic
		Division 2— linguoversion of mandibular teeth.	Class II, Division 2	Retrognathic
Mesiocclusion	Buccal groove of the mandibular first permanent molar is mesial to mesiobuccal cusp of maxillary first permanent molar.	Mandibular teeth mesial to normal position.	Class III	Prognathic

Class II—Distocclusion

In a Class II relationship, the mandibular first permanent molar and canine are distal—that is, more posterior, by at least the width of a premolar, than the ideal position. Even when the molars are in a more distal position, other deviations can occur, creating two divisions within a Class II occlusion.

Division I. A protrusion of incisors or overjet; overbite, crowding, or a labial inclination of the maxillary incisors.

Division II. A protrusion of the maxillary lateral incisors; a retrusion of the maxillary central incisors.

A Class II malocclusion can occur on one side of the arch while the other side remains a Class I.

Class III—Mesiocclusion

In a Class III relationship, the permanent mandibular first molar and canine are mesial—that is, more anterior, by at least the width of a premolar, than the normal position. When the molars are more mesially located, there are other conditions that can also occur such as an anterior crossbite or edge-to-edge contact of the anterior teeth.

Although it was developed almost 100 years ago, Angle's classification remains the most popular method of classifying malocclusions today. However, this classification is based solely on clinical examination. With the development of other techniques to diagnose true malocclusions, principally that of cephalometric radiographs and analyses, today's definitions of malocclusions go far beyond the relationship of maxillary and mandibular teeth to each other. These include the mesiodistal and anterior–posterior relationship of the mandible and maxilla to each other and to some fixed reference point, namely, the cranial bone. Today, the classification of malocclusion is more complicated as it considers not only dental anomalies but also skeletal and developmental deviations, together with soft tissue and nasal and oral airway influences.

RELATED TERMS

Profiles: **Mesognathic** describes the normal profile (Table 15-2). When the mandible protrudes it is called **prognathic** (Table 15-2); when the mandible retrudes it is called **retrognathic** (Table 15-2).

Centric Occlusion: This refers to the relationship of the occlusal surfaces of one arch to those in the opposing arch. The posterior teeth are closed; the anterior teeth have a very light or no contact.

Centric Relation: This refers to the most retruded position of the condyle in the mandibular fossa.

Mastication: Mastication is the process whereby food is chewed. Food is chewed first on one side of the mouth and then shifted to the other side. The posterior teeth, with assistance of the cheeks, tongue, and lips, perform the major portion of this work.

Functional Malocclusion: This is an occlusal deviation created by habits or muscular dysfunctions. Certain habits such as thumbsucking or reverse or deviant swallowing may cause a malocclusion depending on the intensity, duration, and/or age at which they occur.

Missing Teeth: Premature loss of primary teeth, missing permanent teeth, or supernumerary teeth can also contribute to a malocclusion because they cause adjacent teeth to shift from their normal alignment.

PRIMARY TEETH OCCLUSION

The spacing of the primary teeth plays an important part of the occlusion of the permanent teeth. Proximal contact is needed for the overall integrity of the permanent teeth, but spacing between primary teeth, particularly the anterior teeth, is needed to provide adequate room for larger permanent teeth. This normal spacing between the anterior deciduous teeth is called *primate spacing*.

Although the jaws will grow, the growth may not provide enough width for the permanent teeth. Lack of primate spacing, or crowding of the anterior teeth, may suggest a future orthodontic problem.

The position of the primary second molar is also an important determinant of permanent tooth alignment. If the second molars are in a Class I position, the permanent teeth will usually be guided into a Class I position. The positioning of the primary second molars is then referred to as *Class I—mesial step* (Figure 15-7).

A.

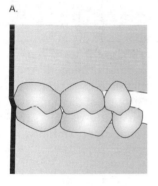

Straight (Flush) Terminal Plane

The distal surfaces of the second primary molars are on the same vertical plane. A moderate number of children have this relationship.

B.

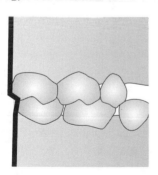

Mesial Step

The distal surface of the mandibular molar is mesial to that of the maxillary molar, thereby forming a mesial step. Most children have this relationship.

C.

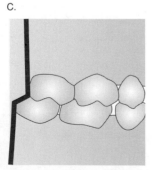

Distal Step

The distal surface of the mandibular molar is distal to that of the maxillary molar, thereby forming a distal step. Few children have this relationship.

FIGURE 15-7
Occlusion of the primary teeth

Often the primary molars will show a cusp-to-cusp (end-to-end) relationship called *terminal plane* (Figure 15-7). An actual end-to-end relationship between the second primary molars is also considered Class I. If the primary molars guide the permanent molars into position, a malocclusion may be seem likely but, in fact, often does not occur. Extra space is provided in the area of the primary molars, allowing for a mesial shift of the permanent mandibular first molars. The primary second molars are wider mesiodistally than the premolars that will replace them, and there is a primate space between the primary canine and first molar. With these two factors and more growth in the arch between ages 8 and 9, a Class I relationship can occur.

SUMMARY

Occlusion occurs when the maxillary and mandibular teeth are in contact in any functional relationship. Ideal occlusion occurs when the teeth conform to a specific pattern of contacts. To simplify the study of occlusion, Angle's classification is frequently used to describe the relationship of first molars and canines. Deviations in the position of teeth or groups of teeth provide a basic understanding of occlusion, but a thorough study of this subject would include all the factors involved in the development, stability, and function of the masticatory system.

WORKSHEET

A. *Using the following illustrations of the maxillary incisor as a guide, draw the mandibular incisor in the appropriate position as labeled.*

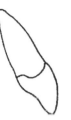

Normal

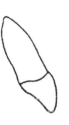

Openbite

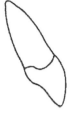

Overbite

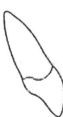

Overjet

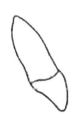

Crossbite

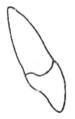

Edge-to-Edge

Form and Function

Proximal Contact Areas
Interproximal Spaces
Embrasures
Compensating Curvatures

OBJECTIVES

- Describe proximal contact areas, interproximal spaces, and embrasures, and understand their importance to the function and integrity of the masticatory system.
- Define Curve of Spee and Curve of Wilson.
- Complete the worksheet at the end of the chapter.

In order for the teeth to cut and masticate food, their appropriate position in the arch must be maintained. Correct positioning is also necessary to assist in the protection of the supporting structures, which in turn sustain the teeth so that they can function properly. Form and function are concerned with how both the position and shape of the teeth enable them to function.

The entire topic of tooth form and function is considerably broad, covering all the conditions that affect tooth alignment in the arches. *Wheeler's Dental Anatomy, Physiology and Occlusion*, by M. Ash, includes nine aspects in the study of this topic:

1. The development of occlusion.
2. Dental arch form.
3. Compensating curvatures and planes of the dental arches.
4. Angulation of the individual teeth in relation to various planes.
5. Functional form of the teeth at their incisal and occlusal thirds.
6. Facial relations of each tooth in one arch to its antagonist(s) in the opposing arch in centric occlusion.
7. Occlusal contact and intercusp relations of all teeth of one arch with those in the opposing arch in centric occlusion.
8. Occlusal contact and intercusp relations of all teeth during various functional mandibular movements.
9. Neurobehavioral aspects of occlusion.

An entire study of occlusion would be necessary to thoroughly cover these topics. Only a basic introduction to form and function is given in this chapter, covering those aspects that are most useful to the dental assistant. This includes the topics of proximal contact areas, interproximal space, and embrasures. Further study is recommended when considering oromotor functions, prosthetic rehabilitation, or orthodontics.

PROXIMAL CONTACT AREAS

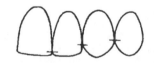

FIGURE 16-1
Contact areas

The **proximal contact area** is a small spot on the mesial and distal surface of each tooth that touches, or contacts, the proximal tooth. Every tooth, except the last molars in each arch, has both a distal and mesial contact area. Contact areas are shown on Figure 16-1 by horizontal lines. This area is generally the widest point on the crown of the tooth.

Contact areas of the anterior teeth are located more incisally that those of the posterior teeth. A review of the individual teeth shows the contact areas of the posterior teeth located at about the middle of the tooth.

Function of Contact Areas

Proper contact between teeth prevents food from packing between them, thus protecting the gingiva from any irritation that could result from food that is lodged between the teeth. In addition, contact areas stabilize the teeth in the arch by providing mutual support.

INTERPROXIMAL SPACES

The **interproximal space** is an area between each tooth normally filled with the interdental papilla. Its boundaries form a triangle with the sides of the proximal surfaces of the teeth; the base in the alveolar crest and the apex is the contact area (Figure 16-2).

Function of the Interproximal Space

Appropriate width between each tooth (the base of the triangle) is important to provide enough space for periodontal structures; to allow ample bone between each tooth for adequate support; and to maintain the level of the gingival tissue (Figure 16-3).

EMBRASURES

Any curvature, either toward or away from the contact area, is an **embrasure** (Figure 16-4). Embrasures are located on the incisal, occlusal, lingual, or facial surface and are often referred to as spillways because they assist the food in "spilling" away from the tooth.

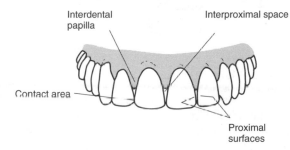

Interdental papilla

Interproximal space

Contact area

Proximal surfaces

FIGURE 16-2
Proximal surfaces and contact areas

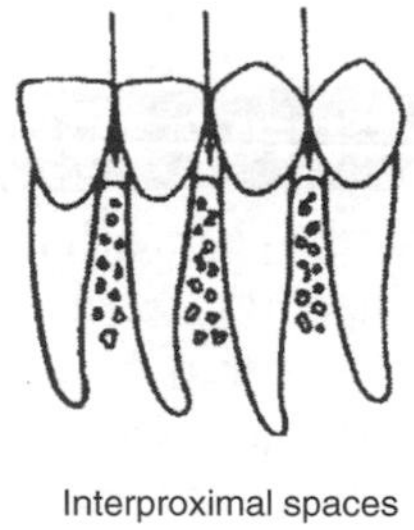

Interproximal spaces

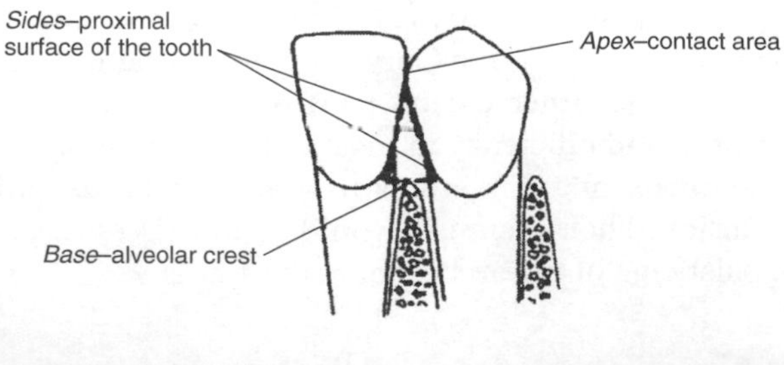

Sides–proximal surface of the tooth

Apex–contact area

Base–alveolar crest

FIGURE 16-3
The boundaries of the interproximal space form a triangle

Occlusal embrasure

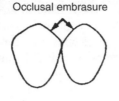

Facial view

Curve of Spee

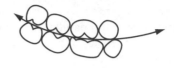

Facial view

Lingual embrasure

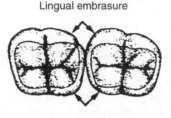

Facial embrasure

Curve of Wilson

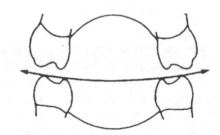

FIGURE 16-4
Embrasures

FIGURE 16-5
The Curve of Spee and the Curve of Wilson—frontal views

Function of the Embrasures

The embrasures or spillways act as an escapement for food so that it does not cling to the teeth or get forced into the interproximal spaces. In this way, embrasures act to assist in cleansing the tooth and to protect the gingival tissue from being irritated by keeping the food away from it.

COMPENSATING CURVATURES

The occlusal plane of the tooth is a line that extends from the incisal edge of the central incisors to the distal buccal cusp of the second molar. Von Spee first noted that this line, when viewed from a point opposite the first molars, forms a curve when the teeth have erupted and are in normal alignment. This curve, which is concave toward the mandible, is the Curve of Spee, named after Von Spee, who first defined it (Figure 16-5).

When the arches are viewed from a frontal position, another curvature is seen extending from the cusp tip of the right molar to the cusp tip of the left molar. This concave curvature is the Curve of Wilson (again, see Figure 16-4).

Together, these and other **compensating curvatures** of the arches account for strength and efficiency in mastication and assist in the stability of the teeth. Compensating curvatures have no special use other than to help define occlusion. Their main use would be in the construction of dentures or in the balancing of the arches for orthodontia.

SUMMARY

Although many factors affect the form and function of the teeth, only three of these are examined here in order to provide a basic understanding of the importance of the appropriate positioning of each tooth in the arch. Those examined are proper proximal contact areas, which prevent food from packing between the teeth; embrasures, which act as a spillway so that food does not cling to the teeth; and interproximal spacing, which allows adequate space for the periodontal structures to support the teeth.

WORKSHEET

A. Complete the following questions about contact areas.

1. Tooth surfaces that are adjacent to or facing each other are called proximal surfaces. The proximal surfaces are the _____ and _____ surfaces of each tooth.

2. The contact area is that area of the proximal surface that touches the adjacent area. Each tooth contacts its adjacent tooth on the proximal surface.

   Each tooth has two contact areas except the last molar, which has no contacting tooth on the distal.

   Mesial surfaces contact distal surfaces with the exception of the central incisors, where two mesial surfaces meet.

   Place a line on the following figure to represent the location of the contact areas.

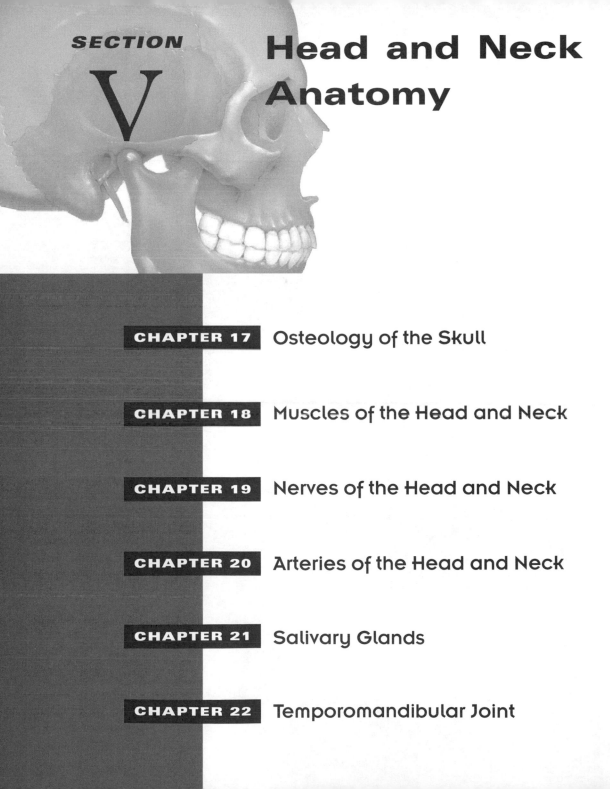

SECTION V

Head and Neck Anatomy

Osteology of the Skull

Neurocranium
Viscerocranium
Maxilla
Mandible
Hyoid bone

OBJECTIVES

- Identify the location of the cranial and facial bones, noted in italics in the chapter.
- Identify the location of the anatomic landmarks on the cranial and facial bones.
- Identify the following foramina or canals: hypoglossal canal, supraorbital, stylomastoid, carotid canal, jugular, rotundum, ovale, foramen magnum, spinosum, lacerum, greater and lesser palantine, incisive.
- Identify the location of the anatomic landmarks on the mandible and maxilla, noted in italics in the chapter.
- Complete the worksheet at the end of the chapter.

NEUROCRANIUM

There are 22 bones that make up the skull. The **neurocranium** is the portion of the cranium that houses and protects the brain. It is made up of the following 8 bones (Figures 17-1 through 17-5):

Single Bones	Paired (Right and Left) Bones
Occipital	Parietal
Sphenoid	Temporal
Ethmoid	
Frontal	

This chapter introduces several new terms. A **suture** is a jagged line where bones join. A **foramen** is a short opening through bone, and a **canal** is a long opening through bone. Nerves and blood vessels travel through canals and foramina.

Occipital Bone

The *occipital bone* forms the posterior aspect of the skull. It articulates or joins with the atlas, or first cervical vertebra, by way of the occipital condyles. These condyles are located on either side of the *foramen magnum*, the large opening through which the spinal cord passes (Figure 17-4).

From an internal view, the occipital bone is divided into four fossae, which house lobes of the brain. The *hypoglossal canals* are located on either side of the foramen magnum. The hypoglossal nerve, an important nerve in dentistry, passes through the hypoglossal canal (Figure 17-5).

Frontal Bone

This bone forms the forehead and anterior aspect of the skull (Figures 17-1 through 17-3). There are four sutures that outline or delineate this bone.

1. *Coronal suture*—joins the frontal and parietal bones
2. *Sagittal suture*—connects the parietal bones
3. *Lambdoidal suture*—joins the occipital and parietal bones
4. *Squamous suture*—connects the parietal and temporal bones

The prominent area of the forehead is known as the *frontal eminence*. The *glabella* is the flattened area between the eyebrows. A *superciliary ridge* is located above each eyebrow. On the superior margin of the orbit (eye) is the *supraorbital foramen* through which passes the supraorbital nerve and artery.

Bones of the Orbit

Six bones make up each orbit: sphenoid, ethmoid, lacrimal, frontal, zygomatic, and maxilla (Figures 17-1 and 17-6). The *optic foramen* is the opening for the optic nerve and ophthalmic artery. Through the *superior orbital fissure*, the oculomotor (III), trochlear (IV), ophthalmic branch of the trigeminal (V), and the abducent (VI) nerves enter the orbit. The *inferior orbital fissure* is the entrance to the orbit for the infraorbital nerve.

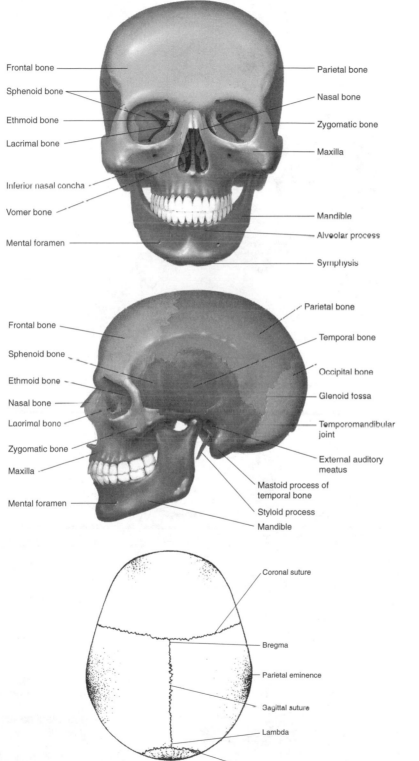

Frontal bone
Sphenoid bone
Ethmoid bone
Lacrimal bone
Inferior nasal concha
Vomer bone
Mental foramen

Parietal bone
Nasal bone
Zygomatic bone
Maxilla
Mandible
Alveolar process
Symphysis

FIGURE 17-1
Skull—anterior aspect

Frontal bone
Sphenoid bone
Ethmoid bone
Nasal bone
Lacrimal bone
Zygomatic bone
Maxilla
Mental foramen

Parietal bone
Temporal bone
Occipital bone
Glenoid fossa
Temporomandibular joint
External auditory meatus
Mastoid process of temporal bone
Styloid process
Mandible

FIGURE 17-2
Skull—lateral aspect

Coronal suture
Bregma
Parietal eminence
Sagittal suture
Lambda
Lambdoidal suture

FIGURE 17-3
Sutures of the skull

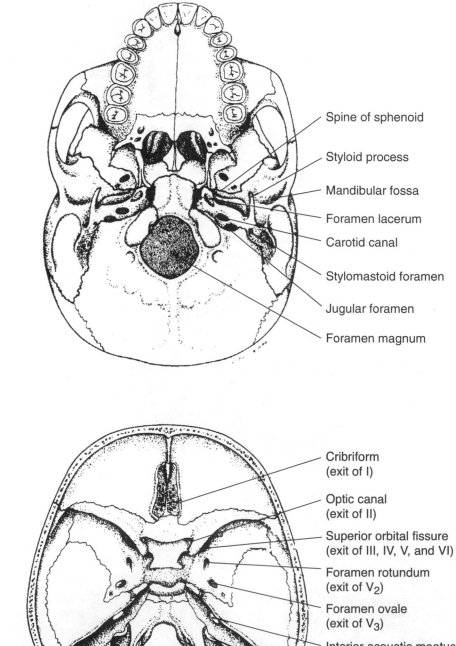

Spine of sphenoid

Styloid process

Mandibular fossa

Foramen lacerum

Carotid canal

Stylomastoid foramen

Jugular foramen

Foramen magnum

FIGURE 17-4
Skull—inferior aspect

Cribriform
(exit of I)

Optic canal
(exit of II)

Superior orbital fissure
(exit of III, IV, V, and VI)

Foramen rotundum
(exit of V_2)

Foramen ovale
(exit of V_3)

Interior acoustic meatus
(exit of VII and VIII)

Jugular foramen
(exit of IX, X, and XI)

Hypoglossal canal
(exit of XII)

FIGURE 17-5
Skull—internal aspect,
showing exit sites of the
cranial nerves

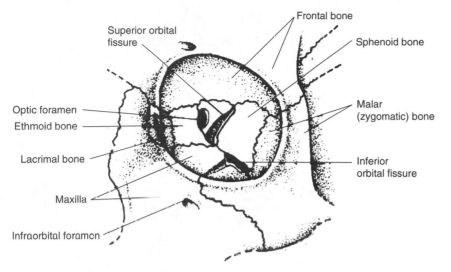

FIGURE 17-6
Bones of the left orbit

Parietal Bones

The *parietal bones* have two curving lines, the superior and inferior temporal lines (Figures 17-1, 17-2, and 17-3). These lines serve as the attachment for the temporalis muscle, a muscle of mastication.

Temporal Bones

The *temporal bones* consist of three parts: the squamous, which is the flattened, fan-shaped portion; the petrous; and the tympanic, which encloses the essential hearing organs (Figure 17-2). The temporal bones have several portions:

- the *zygomatic process*, which extends out to form the zygomatic arch
- the *mandibular (glenoid) fossa*, into which the mandible articulates
- the *articular eminence* or tubercle, a "V"-shaped projection located in front of the glenoid fossa (Figure 17-7)

The *external auditory (acoustic) meatus*, located in the tympanic portion, is the opening for the outer ear. Posterior to this meatus is a rounded prominence known as the *mastoid process* (Figure 17-2). This structure is hollowed out by air cells that communicate with the middle ear. A pointed spicule of bone, the *styloid process*, serves as a muscle and ligament attachment. A small foramen, the *stylomastoid foramen*, is located between the styloid and mastoid processes. This is the opening through which the facial nerve (VII) exits the skull (Figure 17-4).

Just lateral to the occipital condyles and between the petrous portions of the temporal bone is the *jugular foramen*, a large opening through which the internal jugular vein, glossopharyngeal (IV), vagus (X), and (spinal) accessory (XI) nerves exit the skull. The *carotid canal* opening for the internal carotid artery is located in front of the jugular foramen (Figure 17-4).

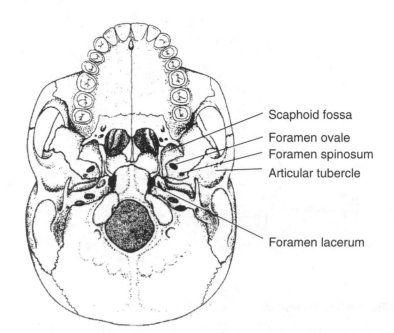

Scaphoid fossa
Foramen ovale
Foramen spinosum
Articular tubercle

Foramen lacerum

FIGURE 17-7
Skull—inferior aspect, showing foramina

Ethmoid Bone

This bone forms a part of the nasal cavity, nasal septum, and orbit. It is located anteriorly at the base of the cranium and is made up of a perpendicular or *cribiform plate*. The cribiform plate is perforated to allow olfactory nerves (relating to the sense of smell) to pass between the brain and nose. The ethmoid bone can be considered a part of either the neurocranium or viscerocranium. For our purposes, we will consider it a portion of the neurocranium.

Sphenoid Bone

This bone looks like a bat with a body, two greater wings and two lesser wings (Figure 17-8). It articulates with *all* the bones that form the cranium. From each greater wing (resembling a butterfly wing), a *pterygoid process* descends. Each pterygoid process (Figure 17-8) is made up of:

- a flattened, *lateral plate* (outside)
- a thinner, *medial plate* (inside)
- a *pterygoid (scaphoid) fossa*—depression between the medial and lateral plates
- a *pterygoid hamulus*—a pointed process that curves outward from the lower (free) end of the medial plate

A depression seen on the surface of the sphenoid bone houses the *pituitary gland*. This depression is known as the *sella turcica* (Figure 17-9).

Three foramina can be seen on the sphenoid bone from the internal aspect. The *foramen rotundum* transmits the maxillary division of the trigeminal nerve (V_2). Through the *foramen ovale*, the mandibular division of the

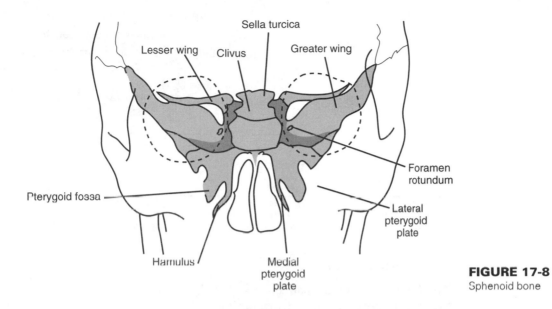

FIGURE 17-8
Sphenoid bone

trigeminal nerve (V_3) passes (Figure 17-7). The *foramen spinosum* (Figure 17-6) transmits the middle meningeal artery to the brain. Next to the foramen ovale is the *foramen lacerum* (Figure 17-7), a channel through which the internal carotid artery travels. In a living human being, the foramen lacerum is covered by a layer of cartilage (Figure 17-7).

VISCEROCRANIUM

There are fourteen bones that make up the **viscerocranium** of the facial skeleton, which gives us our appearance.

Single Bones	Paired (Right and Left) Bones
Mandible	Zygomatic
Vomer	Maxillae
	Nasal
	Lacrimal
	Palatine
	Inferior nasal concha

Zygomatic Bones (Cheek Bones)

The *zygomatic* (singular: *zygoma*) *bones* form the cheeks.

Vomer

The *vomer* forms the posterior and inferior part of the nasal septum (Figure 17-9). The ethmoid bone forms the anterior portion of the nasal septum.

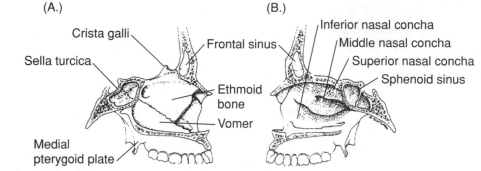

(A.) (B.)

Crista galli — Frontal sinus — Inferior nasal concha — Middle nasal concha — Superior nasal concha — Sphenoid sinus

Sella turcica —

Ethmoid bone

Vomer

Medial pterygoid plate

FIGURE 17-9
Bony nasal septum and cavity: (A) sagittal section showing the bony nasal septum, (B) nasal cavity with nasal septum removed

Nasal Bones

These oblong bones form the bridge of the nose (Figures 17-1 and 17-2).

Lacrimal Bones

The *lacrimal bones* are small and fragile (Figure 17-6). They are located at the anterior portion of the medial orbital wall.

Inferior Nasal Concha

The *inferior nasal concha* lies in the nasal cavity and articulates with the maxilla. The superior and middle nasal conchae are processes of the ethmoid bone; however, the inferior nasal concha is formed as a separate bone (Figure 17-9).

Palatine Bones

Each *palatine bone* is made up of a horizontal plate, which forms the hard palate, and a vertical plate. Two foramina are located in the hard palate. The *greater palatine foramen* is a large opening for the greater palatine nerve and artery. The *lesser palatine foramen* is a small foramen located posterior to the greater palatine foramen. It transmits the lesser palatine nerve and artery (Figure 17-10).

MAXILLA

The *maxilla* is made up of two portions joined by a median suture. It consists of a body and four processes. The *frontal process* and *zygomatic (malar) process* join the frontal and zygomatic bones. The *alveolar process* surrounds and supports the maxillary teeth, and the *palatine process* forms the major portion of the hard palate.

The body of the maxilla contains the *canine eminence*, an elevation of bone over the canine root. The infraorbital nerve exits onto the face through the *infraorbital foramen* just below the inferior margin of the orbit (Figure 17-1). The *maxillary sinus* is the largest of the paranasal sinuses and is

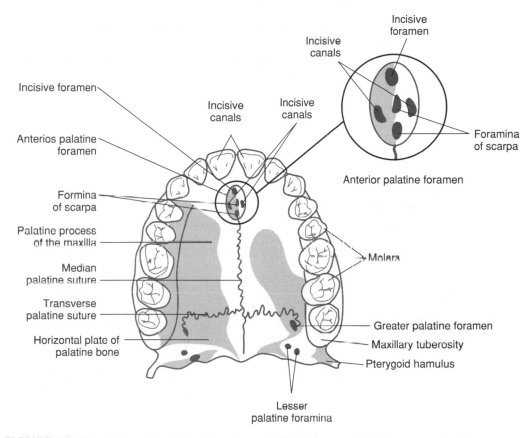

FIGURE 17-10
Maxilla and palatine bones

located within the maxilla above the roots of the maxillary posterior teeth. Posterior to the maxillary third molars is a bulging of bone known as the *maxillary tuberosity* (Figure 17-10).

From an interior view, the *incisive (nasopalatine) foramen* can be seen. It is located on the midline, just behind the maxillary central incisors. It is the opening for the nasopalatine nerve to innervate the hard palate in the maxillary anterior region. It is covered by the incisive papillae (Figure 17-10). The *median palatine suture* marks the articulation of the right and left palatine process. The *transverse palatine suture* is the articulation between the palatine process and the horizontal plates of the palatine bones (Figure 17-10).

MANDIBLE

This is a horseshoe-shaped bone that is made up of a horizontal *body* with right and left vertical *rami* (singular: *ramus*). There is one body and two rami. Each ramus has:

- a *condyle*—a rounded knob that joins with the mandibular (glenoid) fossa
- a *coronoid process*—a pointed, flat projection onto which the temporalis muscle inserts
- a *coronoid*, *mandibular*, or *sigmoid notch*—the curved notch between the condyle and coronoid process (Figures 17-11 and 17-12)

The condyle is attached to the ramus by a thin neck. A triangular depression below the condyle is known as the *pterygoid fovea* to which the lateral pterygoid muscle attaches (Figure 17-11). The *mental protuberance* is the tip of the chin. The *mental foramen* is located on the external surface of the mandible near the apex of the mandibular second premolar. It is the exit point where the mental nerve and vessels branch from the inferior alveolar nerve. A line that extends from the mental foramen along the external surface of the body is known as the *external oblique line* (Figure 17-11).

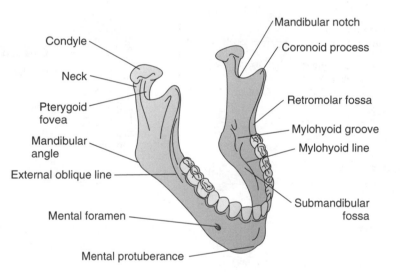

FIGURE 17-11
Mandible—external view

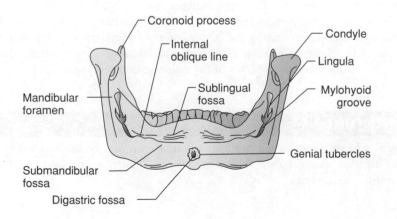

FIGURE 17-12
Mandible—internal view

Internal Surface. On the internal surface of the mandible, the *internal oblique line* can be seen. It runs from the molar region to the midline. It is also known as the *mylohyoid ridge or line* and is the attachment for the mylohyoid muscle. *Genial tubercles or spines,* small projections of bone located on either side of the midline (Figure 17-12), are the site of attachment for the genioglossus and geniohyoid muscles.

The *submandibular fossa* contains the submandibular gland and is located in the premolar and molar region below the mylohyoid line. The sublingual fossa is located on either side of the genial tubercles. The sublingual glands are housed here (Figure 17-12).

The *retromolar fossa* is a triangular area of bone distal to the mandibular third molar (Figure 17-11). The *mandibular foramen* is a large opening located in the center of the ramus. It is the opening into the mandibular canal through which passes the inferior alveolar nerve and artery (Figures 17-10, 17-11, and 17-12). Superior to the mandibular foramen is the *lingual,* a small bony projection which protects the foramen. The *mylohyoid groove* may be visible leading away from the mandibular foramen (Figure 17-12).

HYOID BONE

The hyoid bone is suspended in the neck and is an attachment point for neck and tongue muscles. It is made up of a body and two pairs of horns, the greater cornu and lesser cornu (Figure 17-13). It is horseshoe-shaped and does not articulate with other bones.

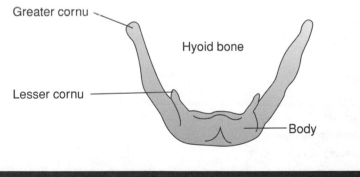

Greater cornu

Hyoid bone

Lesser cornu

Body

FIGURE 17-13
Hyoid bone—anterior view

SUMMARY

The skeleton of the skull is divided into two groups: (1) the neurocranium, 22 bones that make up the skull, and (2) the viscerocranium, 14 bones that make up the face.

Included in the neurocranium are (1) the occipital bone, which forms the posterior aspect of the skull; (2) the frontal bone, which forms the forehead and anterior aspect of the skull; (3) the ethmoid bone, which forms the nasal cavity, nasal septum, and orbit; (4) the sphenoid, ethmoid, lacrimal, frontal, zygomatic, and maxilla, which make up the bones of the orbit; (5) the parietal bones, which form the sides of the skull; and (6) the temporal bones, which house the hearing organs and help to make up the temporo-mandibular joint.

Included in the viscerocranium are (1) the zygomatic bones, which form the cheek; (2) the nasal bones, which form the bridge of the nose; (3) the lacrimal bones; (4) the inferior nasal concha, which lies in the nasal cavity and articulates with the maxilla; (5) the palatine bones, which form the hard palate; (6) the maxilla, which forms the upper jaw; (7) the mandible, which forms the lower jaw; and (8) the vomer, which forms the posterior and inferior part of the nasal septum.

In addition, the hyoid bone, which does not articulate with other bones, is located in the skull. It serves as an attachment for the tongue and neck muscles.

WORKSHEET

A. *Define the following terms.*

foramen

canal

suture

B. *Using a human skull:*

1. Locate the following bones:

occipital

frontal

parietal

temporal

sphenoid

ethmoid

zygomatic

nasal

lacrimal

inferior nasal concha

palatine

2. Locate the following structures on the sphenoid bone.

lateral plate

medial plate

pterygoid fossa

pterygoid hamulus

3. **Locate the following structures on the maxilla.**
    canine eminence
    infraorbital foramen
    maxillary tuberosity
    incisive foramen
    median palatine suture
    transverse palatine suture
    greater palatine foramen
    lesser palatine foramen

4. **Locate the following structures on the mandible.**
    body
    ramus
    condyle
    coronoid process
    pterygoid fovea
    mental protuberance
    mental foramen
    external oblique line
    internal oblique line
    genial tubercles
    submandibular fossa
    sublingual fossa
    retromolar fossa
    mandibular foramen
    mylohyoid groove
    lingula

CHAPTER 18

Muscles of the Head and Neck

Muscles of Mastication
Suprahyoid Muscles
Infrahyoid Muscles
Muscles of the Tongue
Muscles of Facial Expression
Muscles of the Neck
Muscles of the Soft Palate
Muscles of the Pharynx

OBJECTIVES

- Describe the origin, insertion, and function of the muscles of mastication.
- Classify each muscle of the head and neck according to the group in which it belongs.
- Describe the location and function of the muscles of facial expression, suprahyoid and infrahyoid muscles, and muscles of the tongue, neck, soft palate, and pharynx.
- Describe nerve innervation to the various muscle groups.
- Describe the three stages of swallowing.
- Complete the worksheet at the end of the chapter.

Muscles make movements possible by their contraction. Generally, they are suspended between an **origin**, a fixed structure or end, and an **insertion,** the movable end. Names of the muscles may give information about their origin and insertion. Muscles move in the direction of their origin, a fact that helps explain their motion. The muscles of the head and neck are divided into eight groups:

- Muscles of mastication
- Suprahyoid muscles
- Infrahyoid muscles
- Muscles of the tongue
- Muscles of facial expression
- Muscles of the neck
- Muscles of the soft palate
- Muscles of the pharynx

MUSCLES OF MASTICATION

These muscles elevate, protrude, retrude, or cause lateral movement of the mandible. They work during chewing, or **mastication**—hence their name. They are innervated by the mandibular branch of the trigeminal nerve (V_3). The maxillary artery provides blood supply.

Temporalis

The *temporalis* muscle elevates the jaw (Figure 18-1). This fan-shaped muscle starts from the temporal fossa of the temporal bone. The fibers form an anterior and a posterior portion. The anterior fibers are vertical; the posterior fibers are somewhat horizontal. The muscle inserts onto the coronoid process of the mandible and may also insert in the mandible distal to the mandibular third molar. Elevation of the mandible is accomplished when the entire muscle contracts. The mandible is retruded if any of the posterior fibers contract. It can be palpated above the zygomatic arch.

Masseter

This powerful muscle has both a superficial and a deep origin (Figures 18-1 and 18-2). The superficial fibers begin on the anterior two-thirds of the inferior border of the zygomatic arch. The deep fibers start from the posterior one-third of the zygomatic arch. The insertion of the deeper fibers is at the outside surface of the mandible and coronoid process of the mandible. The superficial fibers insert in the outer surface of the angle of the mandible. Contraction of this muscle causes the mandible to elevate. It is easily observed when the jaws are clenched.

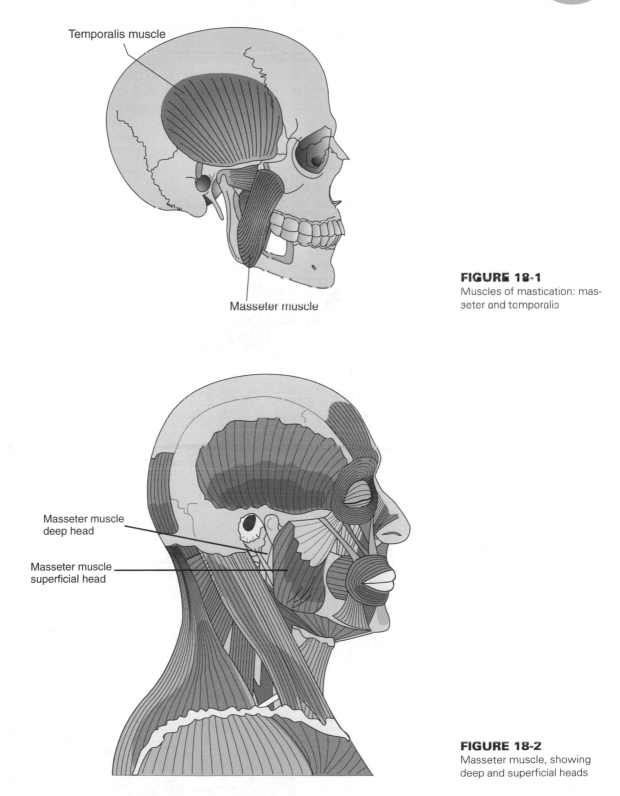

Temporalis muscle

Masseter muscle

FIGURE 18-1
Muscles of mastication: masseter and temporalis

Masseter muscle
deep head

Masseter muscle
superficial head

FIGURE 18-2
Masseter muscle, showing
deep and superficial heads

Medial Pterygoid

This muscle also has both a superficial and a deep origin. The superficial fibers begin at the maxillary tuberosity, while the deep fibers arise from the medial side of the lateral pterygoid plate (Figures 18-3 and 18-4). The muscle inserts on the medial surface of the angle of the mandible. Its function is to elevate the mandible.

Lateral Pterygoid

The smaller, superior head starts from the infratemporal surface of the sphenoid bone and inserts into the articular disc of the temporomandibular joint (Figures 18-3 and 18-4). The larger, inferior head arises from the lat-

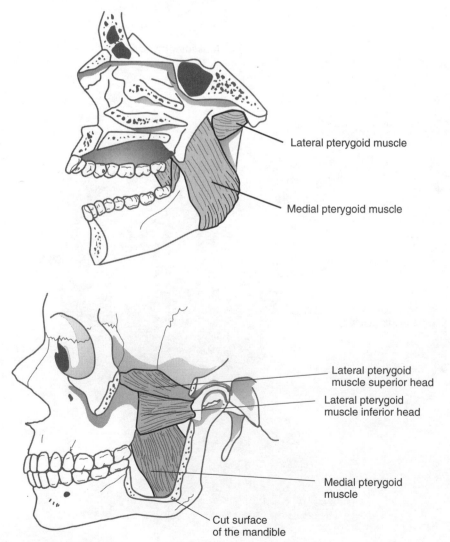

FIGURE 18-3
Medial and lateral pterygoid muscles—internal aspect

Lateral pterygoid muscle

Medial pterygoid muscle

FIGURE 18-4
Pterygoid muscles—lateral aspect (coronoid process and anterior half of ramus of mandible removed)

Lateral pterygoid muscle superior head

Lateral pterygoid muscle inferior head

Medial pterygoid muscle

Cut surface of the mandible

eral surface of the lateral pterygoid plate and inserts in the pterygoid fovea of the mandible. Remember that the origin of the medial pterygoid is the medial surface of the lateral pterygoid plate. If both pterygoid muscles contact, the jaw protrudes. If only one lateral pterygoid muscle contracts, there is a lateral shift of the mandible to the opposite side.

SUPRAHYOID MUSCLES

These muscles are located above the hyoid bone. They are found between the mandible and the hyoid bone and function to lower the mandible or raise the hyoid bone.

Digastic

This slinglike muscle has fibers at either end and is connected in the center by an intermediate tendon or sling (Figures 18-5, 18-6, and 18-7). The anterior belly begins on the digastric fossa of the mandible (the inferior surface of the mandible at the midline) and inserts into the intermediate tendon. The posterior belly starts from the intermediate tendon and inserts on the digastric notch (medial to the mastoid process). The anterior belly is innervated by the mandibular branch of the trigeminal nerve (V_3). The facial nerve (VII)* supplies the posterior belly.

Mylohyoid

This muscle creates the floor of the mouth (Figures 18-5, 18-6, and 18-7). It begins on the mylohyoid line of the mandible and inserts into a raphe at its midline. It is innervated by the mandibular branch of the trigeminal nerve.

Geniohyoid

This muscle arises from the genial tubercles of the mandible and inserts on the hyoid bone (Figure 18-6). It is innervated by the hypoglossal nerve (XII) and is located above the mylohyoid muscle.

Stylohyoid

The origin of this muscle is the styloid process, which its insertion is the hyoid bone. It lies near the posterior belly of the digastric (Figures 18-6 through 18-9). It is innervated by the same branch of the facial nerve that supplies the posterior belly of the digastric.

*Refer to Chapter 19 for nerve designations.

A.

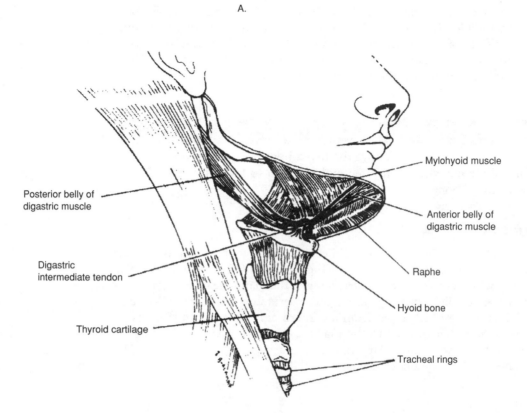

Posterior belly of
digastric muscle

Digastric
intermediate tendon

Thyroid cartilage

Mylohyoid muscle

Anterior belly of
digastric muscle

Raphe

Hyoid bone

Tracheal rings

B.

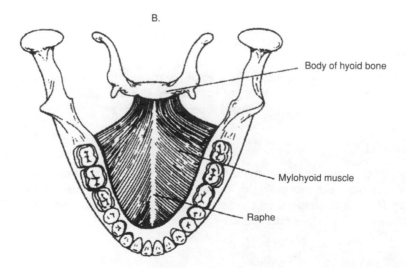

Body of hyoid bone

Mylohyoid muscle

Raphe

FIGURE 18-5
Mylohyoid muscle

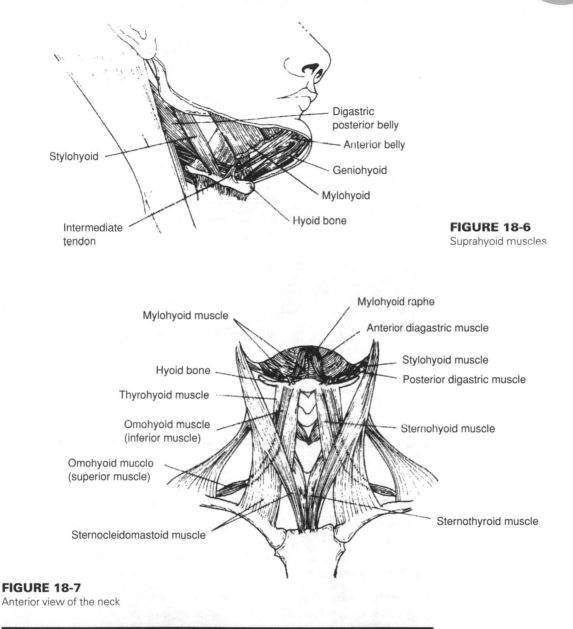

Digastric
posterior belly

Anterior belly

Stylohyoid

Geniohyoid

Mylohyoid

Hyoid bone

Intermediate
tendon

FIGURE 18-6
Suprahyoid muscles

Mylohyoid muscle

Mylohyoid raphe

Anterior diagastric muscle

Hyoid bone

Stylohyoid muscle

Thyrohyoid muscle

Posterior digastric muscle

Omohyoid muscle
(inferior muscle)

Sternohyoid muscle

Omohyoid muscolo
(superior muscle)

Sternocleidomastoid muscle

Sternothyroid muscle

FIGURE 18-7
Anterior view of the neck

INFRAHYOID MUSCLES

These muscles are located below the hyoid bone, in front of the neck. They function to depress the hyoid or fix it in place so the suprahyoid can work. They are innervated by the first, second, and third cervical nerves.

Omohyoid

This muscle has two bellies that are joined by an intermediate tendon (Figures 18-7 and 18-8). The inferior belly comes from the scapula and ends on

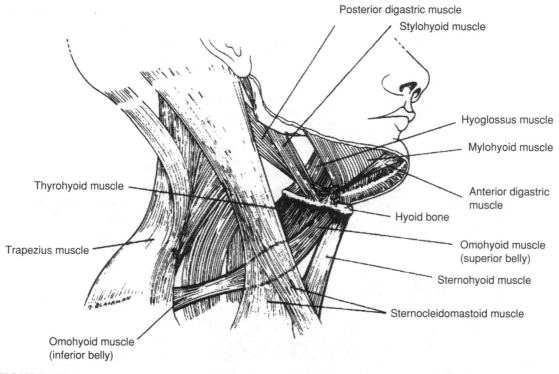

FIGURE 18-8
Lateral view of the neck

the intermediate tendon, while the superior belly originates on the intermediate tendon and inserts on the hyoid bone.

Sternohyoid

The origin of this muscle is the sternum, and its insertion is the hyoid bone (Figures 18-7 and 18-8).

Sternothyroid

This muscle arises from the sternum and inserts on the thyroid cartilage (Figure 18-7). It is located below the sternohyoid.

Thyrohyoid

The *thyrohyoid* originates on the thyroid cartilage and inserts on the hyoid bone (Figure 18-8).

MUSCLES OF THE TONGUE

The muscles of the tongue are divided into two groups, intrinsic and extrinsic. These muscles help the tongue to change its shape and position. Tongue muscles are innervated by the hypoglossal nerve (XII).

Intrinsic Muscles

These muscles lie in and are contained entirely within the tongue. They are responsible for changes in the shape of the tongue and are named for the direction in which they run. These muscles are confluent, so they are not viewed as individual muscles.

Superior Longitudinal

This muscle runs the length of the tongue from anterior to posterior. Located near the top of the tongue, it functions to widen the tongue and turn the tip up.

Inferior Longitudinal

This muscle also runs the length of the tongue from anterior to posterior; however, it lies near the bottom of the tongue. It also widens the tongue, but turns the tip down.

Transverse

This muscle is found on the lateral edges of the tongue. Its function is to make the tongue narrow.

Vertical

This muscle runs from the upper surface to the lower surface of the tongue. It aids in widening the tongue tip.

Extrinsic Muscles

These muscles originate from close structures and insert on or intermingle with intrinsic muscles. They aid in positioning the tongue.

Genioglossus

The origin of this muscle is the genial tubercles, and its insertion is on the tongue and hyoid bone (Figure 18-9). Anterior fibers retract the tongue, and posterior fibers push it forward. This muscle does a majority of work for the tongue.

Hyoglossus

This muscle originates on the hyoid bone and inserts on the side of the tongue. It depresses the tongue and draws the sides down (Figure 18-9).

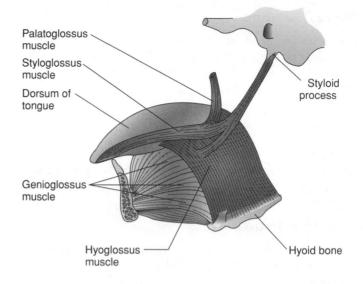

Palatoglossus muscle

Styloglossus muscle

Dorsum of tongue

Styloid process

Genioglossus muscle

Hyoglossus muscle

Hyoid bone

FIGURE 18-9

Extrinsic muscles of the tongue

Styloglossus

This muscle is from the styloid process and has two insertions on the tongue. One head intermingles with the inferior longitudinal and the other joins with the hyoglossus. The styloglossus draws the tongue up and backward.

Palatoglossus

This muscle forms the anterior tonsillar arch (in front of the tonsils). Its origin is the underside of the soft palate and its insertion is the posterior side of the tongue. It is innervated by the pharyngeal plexus, a group of branches from the glossopharyngeal (IX), vagus (X), and spinal accessory (XI) nerves. Its contraction pulls the sides of the tongue faucial up and back, and the soft palate down. It also constricts the pillars.

MUSCLES OF FACIAL EXPRESSION

Contraction of these muscles results in a wide variety of facial expressions. The facial nerve (VII) provides innervation to these muscles. These muscles are symmetric and work in groups.

Muscles of the Scalp

The *occipitofrontalis* (*epicranius*) is made up of two groups, the *frontalis* and *occipitalis* (Figure 18-10). This muscle pulls the scalp forward and backward and raises the eyebrows.

Muscles of the Ears

There are three groups of ear muscles: *anterior auricular*, *posterior auricular*, and *superior auricular* (Figure 18-10). They are respectively located in front

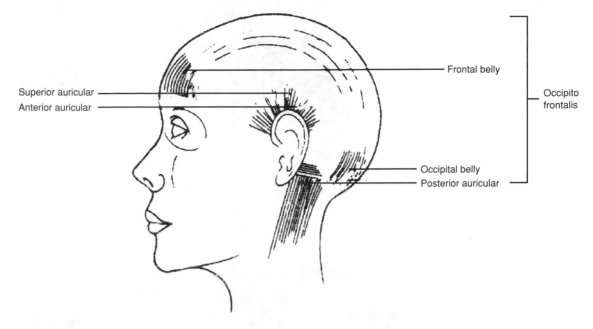

Superior auricular
Anterior auricular
Frontal belly
Occipito frontalis
Occipital belly
Posterior auricular

FIGURE 18-10
Muscles of the scalp and ears

of, behind, and above the ear. These muscles may draw the ear forward and backward or elevate the ear.

Orbicularis Oculi

This muscle encircles the eye. It is divided into orbital and palpebral (eyelid) sections, and it functions to close the eyes.

Procerus

This muscle runs from the bridge of the nose to the eyebrow (Figure 18-11). It pulls the eyebrows downward.

Corrugator

The *corrugator* runs along the eyebrow and inserts on the medial end of the eyebrow (Figure 18-11). It pulls the eyebrow down and in.

Muscles of the Nose

The *nasalis* is divided into two parts: the *compressor nares* and the *dilator nares* (Figure 18-11). The dilator nares cause flaring of the nostrils. The compressor nares close the nostrils.

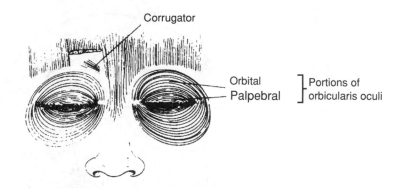

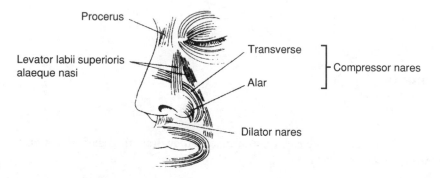

FIGURE 18-11
Muscles of the eye and nose

Muscles of the Mouth

Orbicularis Oris.   This muscle has no skeletal attachment. It encircles the mouth and composes the lips (Figure 18-12). Its function is to close the lips or protrude them. Its fibers interface with other perioral muscles.

Levator Labii Superioris Alaeque Nasi. This tiny muscle inserts on the ala of the nose and runs to the upper lip (Figure 18-13). It raises the upper lip and ala of the nose producing a sneer.

Levator Labii Superioris or Quadratus Labii Superioris. This muscle runs above the mouth and has three heads:

1. *angular*—near the nose
2. *infraorbital*—lower edge of orbit
3. *zygomatic*—zygomatic bone

All three heads insert onto the upper lip and help elevate the upper lip (Figure 18-13).

Zygomatic.   The origin of this muscle is the zygomatic bone, and it inserts into the corner of the mouth or the *modiolus*, an area of intertwining

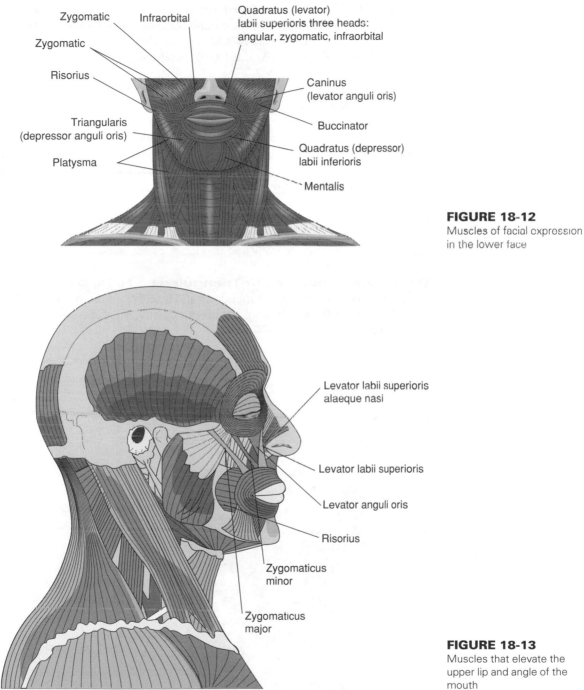

FIGURE 18-12
Muscles of facial expression in the lower face

FIGURE 18-13
Muscles that elevate the upper lip and angle of the mouth

muscles. It elevates the angle of the mouth up and laterally producing a smile. It may be divided into zygomatic major and minor muscles (Figures 18-12 and 18-13).

Levator Anguli Oris or Caninus.   The origin of this muscle is the canine fossa, a depression near the canine roots below the infraorbital foramen. It inserts into the *modiolus* and aids in elevating the corner of the mouth (Figures 18-12, 18-13, and 18-14) producing a smile.

Buccinator.   This muscle forms the cheek (Figure 18-15). It originates from the alveolar process of the mandible, the maxilla, and the pterygomandibular raphe, a fibrous band that runs from the pterygoid hamulus to the mylohyoid line. It blends with the orbicularis oris at the modiolus. The *buccinator* holds the cheek against the teeth and keeps food on the occlusal surfaces during mastication. Because of this function it is considered an accessory muscle to the muscles of mastication.

Risorius.   This muscle originates on the anterior border of the masseter muscle and inserts into the modiolus (Figures 18-12 and 18-13). It pulls the angle of the mouth laterally and produces a wide smile.

Depressor Anguli Oris or Triangularis.   This muscle arises from the external oblique line of the mandible and inserts into the modiolus (Figure 18-12). It pulls the corner of the mouth downward and inward producing a frown.

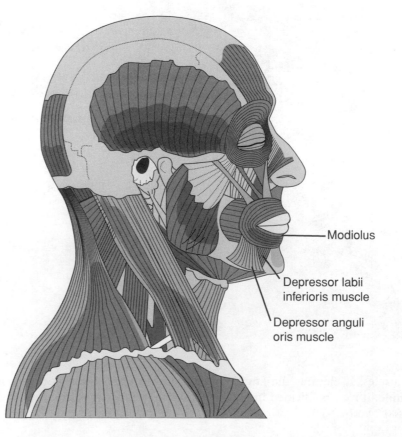

Modiolus

Depressor labii inferioris muscle

Depressor anguli oris muscle

FIGURE 18-14

Muscles that depress the lower lip and angle of the mouth

Depressor Labii Inferioris or Quadratus Labii Inferioris.
This muscle also arises from the external oblique line; however, it inserts
into the skin of the lower lip (Figures 18-12 and 18-14). It functions to pull
the lower lip down and laterally, showing the mandibular anterior teeth.

Mentalis.   This is the only muscle whose fibers run away from the lips
(Figure 18-12). Its origin is a fossa or depression beneath the mandibular
anterior teeth, and it inserts into the skin of the chin. It can raise the skin of
the chin and protrude the lower lip. It often interferes with treatment of
mandibular anterior labial surfaces when contracted.

MUSCLES OF THE NECK

Platysma

The *platysma* is a thin sheet of muscle located just below the skin of the neck
(Figures 18-15 and 18-16). Its origin is the clavicle and shoulder; it travels
upward to insert on the lower border of the mandible as well as on the skin
and muscle of the lower face and mouth. Contraction of this muscle wrinkles
the skin of the chin and neck, and draws the outer part of the lower lip down
and back, producing a grimace. It is innervated by the facial nerve (VII).

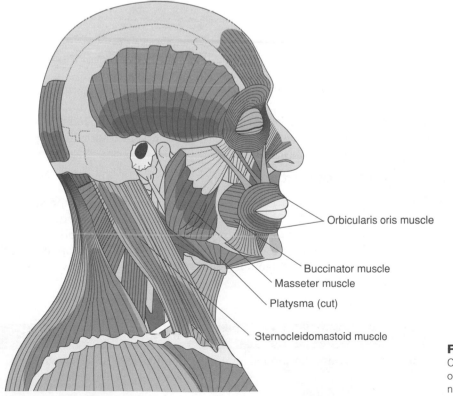

Orbicularis oris muscle

Buccinator muscle
Masseter muscle

Platysma (cut)

Sternocleidomastoid muscle

FIGURE 18-15
Cheek muscles in relation to
other muscles of the face and
neck

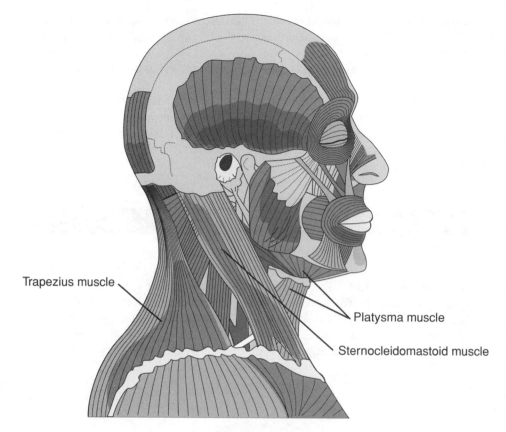

Trapezius muscle

Platysma muscle

Sternocleidomastoid muscle

FIGURE 18-16
Platysma muscle—lateral aspect

Trapezius

This is a large muscle covering the back of the neck, shoulder, and clavicle (Figures 18-8 and 18-16). It originates from the external occipital protuberance and inserts into the clavicle and shoulder. This muscle produces a shoulder shrug. The spinal accessory nerve (XI) provides innervation to this muscle.

Sternocleidomastoid

This prominent muscle arises by two heads, from the top of the sternum and clavicle (Figures 18-7, 18-8, 18-15, and 18-16). The two heads blend together and insert on the mastoid process and the superior nunchal line of the occipital bone. This muscle turns the chin upward to the opposite side when the head is turned laterally. Innervation is provided by the spinal accessory nerve (XI).

MUSCLES OF THE SOFT PALATE

These muscles raise the soft palate during **deglutition**, or swallowing.

Palatoglossus or Palatoglossal

This muscle was discussed previously under "Extrinsic Tongue Muscles." It is associated with both the tongue and the soft palate (Figure 18-17). It forms the anterior tonsillar pillar.

Palatopharyngeal or Palatopharyngeous

This muscle forms the posterior tonsillar pillar (Figures 18-17 and 18-18). Contraction of this muscle causes the pharynx to elevate. It is innervated by the pharyngeal plexus.

Uvula

This small mass of tissue hangs down in the throat from the soft palate (Figure 18-17). Upon contraction, the *uvula* will shorten. Innervation is through the pharyngeal plexus.

Levator Veli Palatini

This muscle originates from the petrous portion of the temporal bone, and it inserts in the soft palate (Figures 18-17 and 18-18). It pulls the soft palate upward and back, and is innervated by the pharyngeal plexus.

Tensor Veli Palatini

This muscle arises from the medial pterygoid plate and auditory tube (Figures 18-17 and 18-18). It turns upward, curves around the pterygoid

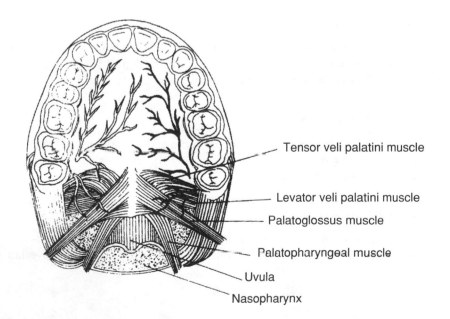

— Tensor veli palatini muscle

— Levator veli palatini muscle

— Palatoglossus muscle

— Palatopharyngeal muscle

— Uvula

Nasopharynx

FIGURE 18-17
Muscles of the soft palate

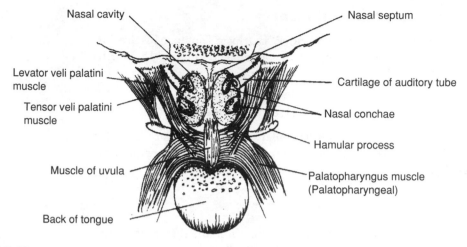

Nasal cavity

Nasal septum

Levator veli palatini muscle

Cartilage of auditory tube

Tensor veli palatini muscle

Nasal conchae

Hamular process

Muscle of uvula

Palatopharyngus muscle (Palatopharyngeal)

Back of tongue

FIGURE 18-18
Posterior view of the muscles of the soft palate

hamulus, and then inserts into the soft palate. It tenses (hence the name) the soft palate by pulling on the lateral sides. It is innervated by the mandibular branch of the trigeminal nerve (V_3).

MUSCLES OF THE PHARYNX

The *pharynx* is a muscular tube. It is made up of three constrictor muscles and three smaller muscles. All the muscles function in deglutition, or swallowing. All constrictors are innervated by the pharyngeal plexus.

Superior Constrictor

The origin of this muscle is the pterygoid hamulus, medial pterygoid plate, pterygomandibular raphe, and the mylohyoid line (Figure 18-19). All three constrictors insert and unite on the *median raphe*.

Middle Constrictor

The greater and lesser horns of the hyoid bone and the stylohyoid ligament are the origins for this muscle (Figure 18-19). It unites with the superior constrictor at the median raphe.

Inferior Constrictor

This muscle arises from the thyroid cartilage of the larynx (Figure 18-19). Its fibers join at the median raphe. Fibers of all three constrictors overlap each other.

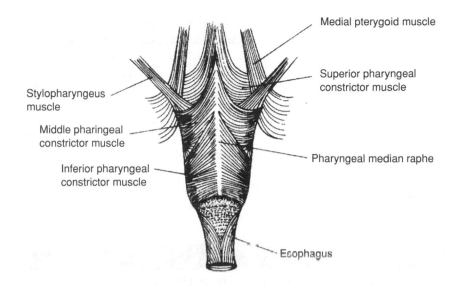

Medial pterygoid muscle

Superior pharyngeal constrictor muscle

Stylopharyngeus muscle

Middle pharingeal constrictor muscle

Inferior pharyngeal constrictor muscle

Pharyngeal median raphe

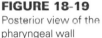

Esophagus

FIGURE 18-19
Posterior view of the pharyngeal wall

Palatopharyngeal

Previously, this muscle was discussed as a muscle of the soft palate. Its function is to elevate the pharynx, so it is also listed here under muscles of the pharynx.

Elevators and Dilators of the Pharynx

Salpingopharyngeal.   The origin of this muscle is the auditory tube. Its fibers blend with the palatopharyngeal muscle. It helps to elevate the pharynx, and it is innervated by the pharyngeal plexus.

Stylopharyngeal.   This muscle arises from the styloid process and inserts on the thyroid cartilage (Figure 18-19). It helps to elevate and dilate the pharynx. Innervation is supplied by the glossopharyngeal nerve (IX).

Deglutition

Swallowing is divided into three stages: *oral*, *pharyngeal*, and *esophageal*.

Oral Stage.   During the oral stage of swallowing, the bolus, a ball of chewed food mixed with saliva, is centered on the tongue. The tongue is then raised up and back and a seal is made between the hard palate and the tongue. The sides of the tongue seal against the teeth and the mucosa of the hard palate. The bolus is moved backward by the intrinsic and extrinsic muscles of the tongue, as well as by the suprahyoid muscles. The muscles of mastication hold the teeth together. The bolus is now positioned onto the posterior tongue. The upward and backward movement of the tongue causes the muscles of the soft palate to elevate the soft palate.

Pharyngeal Stage. The fauces are narrowed by the palatoglossal muscle. The soft palate contacts the posterior pharyngeal wall. The stylopharyngeal and salpingopharyngeal muscles elevate and dilate the pharynx to make room for the bolus that has just entered the pharynx. The superior, middle, and inferior constrictors squeeze the pharynx, propelling the bolus into the lower end of the pharynx.

The thyroid cartilage of the larynx is raised and brought forward by the thyrohyoid muscle and other muscles. The epiglottis protects the larynx from the bolus. The food is then propelled into the upper part of the esophagus.

Esophageal Stage. The bolus is propelled by peristaltic contractions into the stomach.

SUMMARY

The muscles of the head and neck are divided into eight groups: (1) the *muscles of mastication*, including the temporalis, masseter, and medial and lateral pterygoid, which cause the movement of the mandible; (2) the *suprahyoid* muscles, including the digastric, mylohyoid, geniohyoid, and stylohyoid, which cause movement of the lower mandible and raise the hyoid bone; (3) *infrahyoid* muscles, including omohyoid, sternohyoid, sternothyroid, and thyrohyoid, which depress the hyoid bone or hold it in place so the suprahyoids can work; (4) the *muscles of the tongue*, including the various intrinsic muscles, which change the shape of the tongue, and the various extrinsic muscles, which position the tongue; (5) the *muscles of facial expression*, including the various muscles of the scalp, ear, eye, nose, and neck, which control facial expression; (6) the *muscles of the neck*, including the platysma, trapezius, and sternocleidomastoid, which control the movement of the head, chin, neck, and lips; (7) the *muscles of the soft palate*, including the palatoglossal, palatopharyngeal, uvula, and the levator and tensor veli palatini, which raise the soft palate during swallowing; and (8) the *muscles of the pharynx*, including the superior, middle, and inferior constrictors, palatopharyngeal, salpingopharyngeal, and stylopharyngeal, which control swallowing, allowing the elevation and dilation of the pharynx.

WORKSHEET

A. Define the following terms.

origin

insertion

modiolus

deglutition

B. Complete the chart on the muscles of mastication.

Muscle	Origin	Insertion	Function
Masseter			
Temporalis			
Lateral Pterygoid			
Medial Pterygoid			

C. List the steps that occur during each phase of swallowing.

D. Complete the following figures.

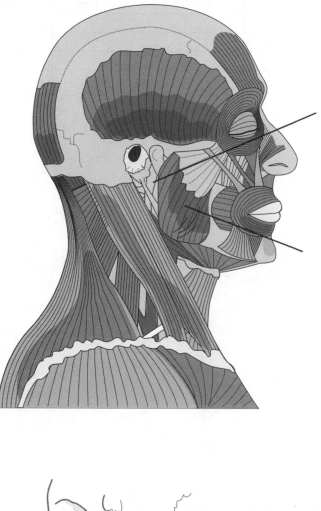

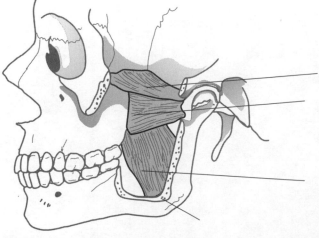

Nerves of the Head and Neck

OBJECTIVES

- List the names and numbers of the cranial nerves.
- Define the following terms: neuron, dendrite, axon, efferent, afferent, somatic, and visceral.
- Describe the central, peripheral, and autonomic nervous systems.
- Differentiate between sympathetic and parasympathetic nerve supply.
- Describe the trigeminal, facial, glossopharyngeal, and hypoglossal nerves according to the following: nerve supply (sensory, motor, or both), structures supplied, teeth supplied, and exit site.
- Describe the nerve supply to each maxillary and mandibular tooth.
- Complete the worksheet at the end of the chapter.

INTRODUCTION

Our nervous system has two parts: the **central nervous system (CNS)** and the **peripheral nervous system (PNS)**. The central nervous system is further classified into two parts: the *brain*, which is housed in the cranium, and the *spinal cord*, which is contained within the vertebral column. The peripheral nervous system is made up of the nerves that travel away from the central nervous system. There are 12 pairs of *cranial* nerves and 31 pairs of *spinal nerves* in the peripheral nervous system. Through the peripheral nervous system, all parts of the body are connected to the central nervous system.

A nerve cell is also known as a *neuron*. A neuron has three parts (Figure 19-1):

1. Cell body
2. Dendrite—a process that conducts impulses toward the cell body. A neuron may have one or many dendrites.
3. Axon—a process that carries impulses away from the cell body. A neuron has only one axon.

Nerves that carry impulses or messages toward the brain are known as **sensory** or **afferent**. Those nerves that carry impulses away from the brain are termed **motor** or **efferent**. **Somatic** nerves supply muscles, while **visceral** nerves provide innervation to the internal organs (viscera).

The **autonomic nervous system** regulates those functions over which we have no conscious control, such as heart rate and respiratory rate. This nervous system is divided into two parts: **sympathetic** and **parasympathetic**.

Usually each organ has sympathetic and parasympathetic nerves supplying it. These systems tend to produce opposite actions.

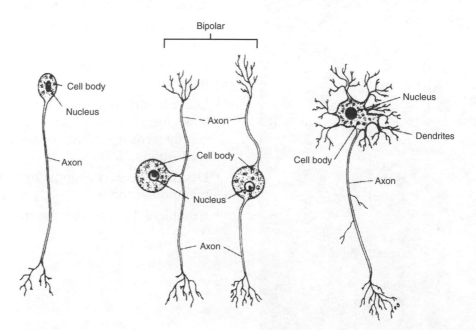

FIGURE 19-1
Shapes of neurons

The sympathetic system functions in response to emergencies. Sympathetic nerves increase respiration, heart rate, and blood flow to muscles. They decrease salivary flow and blood supply to the digestive tract in order that additional blood can be supplied to other muscles. This is often referred to as the "fight or flight" reaction.

The parasympathetic system slows down the heart and respiration; parasympathetic nerves increase blood to the digestive system and salivary glands.

THE CRANIAL NERVES

As mentioned before, there are 12 sets of ("paired") cranial nerves. They provide innervation to the right and left sides of the body, and are designated by Roman numerals. They may be entirely sensory, entirely motor, or a combination of both sensory and motor (mixed). This text concentrates on four cranial nerves that are important for dental auxiliaries: the trigeminal (V), facial (VII), glossopharyngeal (IX), and hypoglossal (XII). The remaining cranial nerves appear in Table 19-1.

THE TRIGEMINAL NERVE (V) (MIXED)

This is the largest cranial nerve and the most important to dental assistants because it provides sensory innervation from the face, scalp, teeth, nose, and mouth. It also distributes motor innervation to the muscles of mastication and provides parasympathetic supply to the salivary and lacrimal glands. Sensory cells are located in the semilunar (gasserian) ganglion found in the petrous portion of the temporal bone. The motor root originates in the pons and joins the mandibular division. The trigeminal nerve has three divisions or branches (Figure 19-2):

1. Ophthalmic nerve (V_1)—entirely afferent
2. Maxillary nerve (V_2)—entirely afferent
3. Mandibular nerve (V_3)—mixed, both afferent and efferent

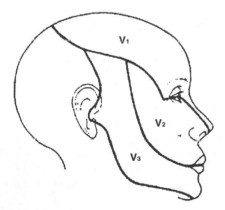

FIGURE 19-2
Area of distribution of the three divisions of the trigeminal nerve

TABLE 19-1   OTHER CRANIAL NERVES

Cranial Nerve	Sensory (S) Motor (M) Both (B)	Function	Exit Site
Olfactory I	S	Sense of smell	Cribiform plate
Optic II	S	Sight	Optic foramen (canal)
Oculomotor III	M	Motor to extrinsic eye muscles (superior and inferior rectus muscles and inferior oblique)	Superior orbital fissure
Trochlear IV	M	Motor to superior oblique eye muscle	Superior orbital fissure
Abducent VI	M	Motor to lateral rectus eye muscle	Superior orbital fissure
Acoustic VII	S	Hearing and balance	Internal acoustic (auditory) meatus
Vagus X	B	Longest cranial nerve. Sensory innervation to ear, pharynx, larynx, bronchi, lungs, heart, esophagus, stomach, intestines, and kidney. Para-sympathetic control of heart rate.Contributes to pharyngeal plexus.	Jugular foramen
(Spinal) Accessory XI	M	Has a cranial and spinal part. Associated with vagus (X) nerve. Contributes to pharyngeal plexus. Motor to trapezius and sternocleidomastoid muscles.	Jugular foramen

The Ophthalmic Nerve

This nerve enters the eye through the *superior orbital fissure* and provides sensory innervation to the eye, nose, lacrimal gland, and skin of the eyelids, forehead, and nose. It has three branches (none of which lead to the oral cavity):

1. *Lacrimal nerve*—innervates the lacrimal glands for tear production and supplies the skin of the upper eyelid.
2. *Frontal nerve*—passes above the eye, dividing into the *supraorbital* and *supratrochlear* nerves. The supraorbital branch supplies the skin of the forehead, scalp, and upper eyelid. The supratrochlear branch supplies the skin of the forehead and upper eyelid (Figure 19-3).
3. *Nasociliary nerve*—runs within the orbit, passes through the ethmoid bone, and reenters the cranium at the cribiform plate of the ethmoid bone. It then passes down into the nose and supplies the inside of the nose and skin on the side of the nose. Its branch, the *infratrochlear nerve*, supplies the medial side of the eyelids and side of the nose.

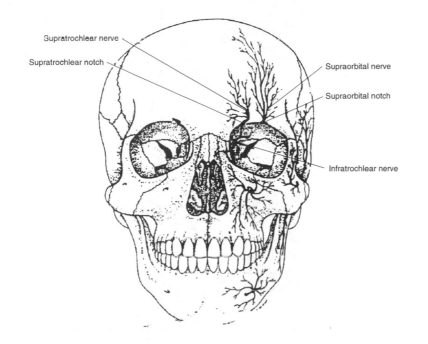

FIGURE 19-3
Branches of the frontal and nasociliary nerves

The Maxillary Nerve (V₂)

The second division of the trigeminal nerve exits the skull through the *foramen rotundum* and passes into the pterygopalatine fossa. In this fossa, the maxillary nerve divides into four branches: *zygomatic, infraorbital, posterior superior alveolar (PSA)*, and *pterygopalatine*.

The Zygomatic Nerve. This nerve enters the eye through the inferior orbital fissure. It has two branches (Figure 19-4):

1. *Zygomaticotemporal*—supplies the skin and side of the forehead
2. *Zygomaticofacial*—supplies the skin of the cheek

The Infraorbital Nerve. This nerve emerges onto the face through the *infraorbital foramen* on the maxilla, but before this nerve exits through the infraorbital foramen it gives off two descending branches (Figures 19-5 and 19-6).

1. *The Middle Superior Alveolar* (MSA) nerve provides innervation to the mesiobuccal root of the maxillary first molar, the maxillary first and second premolars, the adjacent gingiva, and the maxillary sinus. The middle superior alveolar nerve is not always present. If it is not present, innervation to that area is provided by the anterior and posterior superior alveolar nerves (Figures 19 5 and 19-6).
2. *The Anterior Superior Alveolar* (ASA) nerve supplies the maxillary incisor and canine teeth and associated labial gingiva. It also innervates the maxillary sinus (Figures 19-5 and 19-6).

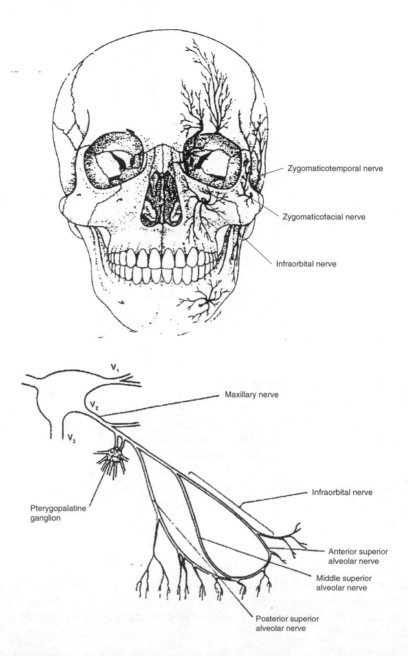

FIGURE 19-4
Branches of the zygomatic
and infraorbital nerves

Zygomaticotemporal nerve

Zygomaticofacial nerve

Infraorbital nerve

Maxillary nerve

Infraorbital nerve

Pterygopalatine
ganglion

Anterior superior
alveolar nerve

Middle superior
alveolar nerve

Posterior superior
alveolar nerve

FIGURE 19-5
Maxillary division of the
trigeminal nerve, showing
branches of the infraorbital
nerve

After the infraorbital nerve emerges onto the face through the infraorbital foramen, it divides into three terminal branches:

3. *Palpebral*—supplies the skin of the lower eyelid
4. *External nasal*—innervates the skin and mucosa of the side of the nose
5. *Superior labial*—supplies the skin and mucosa of the upper lid and labial mucosa

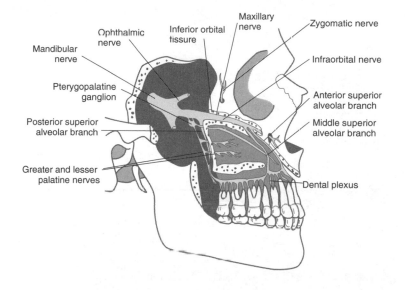

FIGURE 19-6
Branches of the maxillary nerve

Posterior Superior Alveolar (PSA) Nerve.   Before the infraorbital nerve enters the intraorbital groove, it gives off the posterior superior alveolar nerve (Figures 19-5 and 19-6). This nerve crosses the maxillary tuberosity and supplies the maxillary molar teeth, with the exception of the mesiobuccal root and the maxillary first molar, which is innervated by the middle superior alveolar nerve (MSA). The adjacent buccal gingiva and maxillary sinus are also supplied by the posterior superior alveolar nerves.

Pterygopalatine Nerves.   Five branches of the maxillary nerve are given off in the pterygopalatine fossa (Figure 19-7).

1. *Pharyngeal*—supplies the pharynx and pharyngeal mucosa
2. *Greater palatine*—enters the greater palatine foramen (palatine bone) to supply the mucosa of the hard palate and lingual gingiva of the maxillary molars, premolars, and canine teeth
3. *Lesser palatine*—enters the lesser palatine foramen to supply the mucosa of the soft palate and tonsils
4. *Nasopalatine*—passes through the nasopalatine (incisive) foramen of the maxilla to supply the lingual gingiva of the maxillary incisor teeth
5. *Posterior superior lateral nasal*—supplies the middle and superior nasal conchae and the superior nasal septum.

The Mandibular Nerve (V₃)

The mandibular nerve is the largest division of the trigeminal nerve and exits the skull through the *foramen ovale* in the sphenoid bone. It is both afferent and efferent.

After the foramen ovale, the sensory and motor roots of the mandibular nerve unite in a short trunk. The sensory branch gives off the *meningeal nerve*, which passes through the foramen spinosum to supply the meninges.

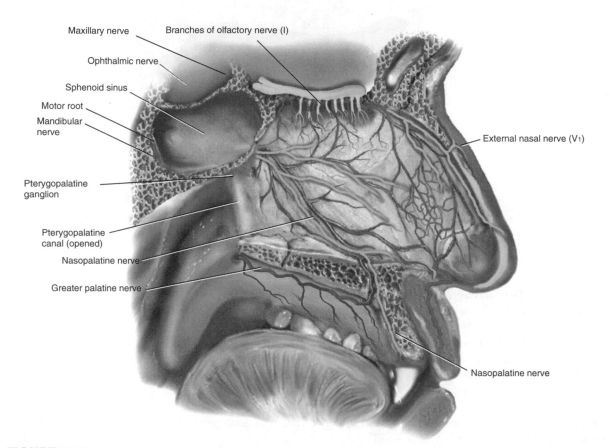

Maxillary nerve

Branches of olfactory nerve (I)

Ophthalmic nerve

Sphenoid sinus

Motor root

Mandibular nerve

External nasal nerve (V1)

Pterygopalatine ganglion

Pterygopalatine canal (opened)

Nasopalatine nerve

Greater palatine nerve

Nasopalatine nerve

FIGURE 19-7
Pterygopalatine nerves

The motor branch distributes nerves to the following muscles: *medial pterygoid*, *tensor tympani*, and *tensor veli palatini*. The mandibular nerve then branches into anterior and posterior divisions.

The Anterior Division.   This division has only one sensory branch; the remaining nerves are all motor to the muscles of mastication (Figure 19-8).

Motor
- *Masseteric nerve*—supplies masseter muscle
- *Anterior and posterior deep temporal nerves*—supply the temporalis muscle
- *Lateral pterygoid nerve*—supplies the lateral pterygoid muscle

Sensory
The *buccal (long buccal) nerve* is the only sensory nerve in the anterior division. It crosses between the two heads of the lateral pterygoid muscle and emerges through the buccinator muscle. It innervates the buccal gingiva of the mandibular molars, the mucosa of the cheek, and the skin of the cheek.

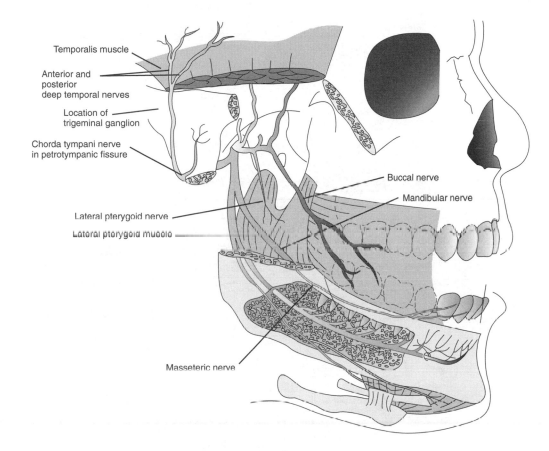

FIGURE 19-8
Anterior division of the mandibular nerve

The Posterior Division.   This division has only one motor branch; the remaining branches are all sensory.

The *auriculotemporal nerve* supplies the skin of the temporal region in front of the ear, the external acoustic (auditory) meatus, and the temporo-mandibular joint (Figure 19-9). After giving off the auriculotemporal nerve, the mandibular nerve divides into two terminal branches.

The *lingual* nerve runs between the medial pterygoid muscle and the mandible. It is joined by the *chorda tympani*, a branch of the facial nerve (VII). Together the lingual and chorda tympani nerves enter the posterior aspect of the mouth and run forward. The *chorda tympani* supplies taste sensation to the anterior two-thirds of the tongue. The lingual nerve enters the floor of the mouth and ventral surface of the tongue. It supplies afferent innervation to the tongue, floor of the mouth, and lingual gingiva of the entire mandibular arch. Remember that the chorda tympani provides taste to the anterior two-thirds of the tongue (Figure 19-10).

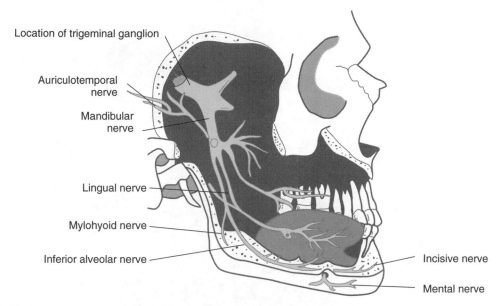

Location of trigeminal ganglion

Auriculotemporal nerve

Mandibular nerve

Lingual nerve

Mylohyoid nerve

Inferior alveolar nerve

Incisive nerve

Mental nerve

FIGURE 19-9

Posterior division of the mandibular nerve

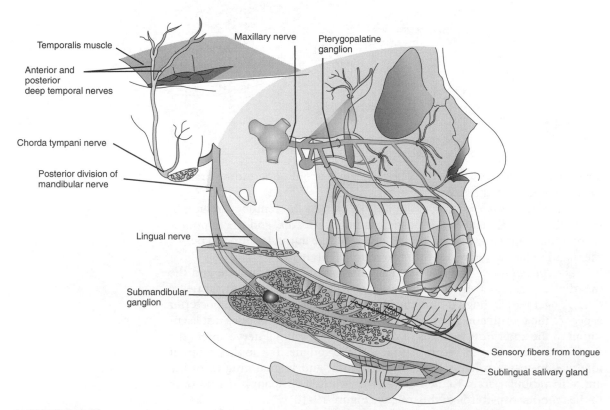

Temporalis muscle

Anterior and posterior deep temporal nerves

Maxillary nerve

Pterygopalatine ganglion

Chorda tympani nerve

Posterior division of mandibular nerve

Lingual nerve

Submandibular ganglion

Sensory fibers from tongue

Sublingual salivary gland

FIGURE 19-10

Branches of the facial nerve

Inferior Alveolar Nerve. This nerve runs parallel with the lingual nerve. It then enters the mandible through the mandibular foramen and continues in the mandibular canal. Before it enters the mandibular foramen, it gives off the *mylohyoid nerve*, the only motor branch in the posterior division. It supplies efferent sensation to the mylohyoid muscle and the anterior belly of the digastric muscle. After giving off the mylohyoid nerve, the inferior alveolar nerve is entirely sensory.

Within the mandibular canal, the inferior alveolar nerve gives off branches to the mandibular molars and premolars. At the *mental foramen*, it divides into the following nerves:

- *Mental nerve*, which supplies the chin and lower lip (Figure 19-9)
- *Incisive nerve*, which supplies the mandibular anterior teeth and labial gingiva (Figure 19-9)

THE FACIAL NERVE (VII)

The facial nerve is both afferent and efferent. It provides molar innervation to all the muscles of facial expression, posterior belly of the digastric muscle, stylohyoid, and stapedius muscle of the middle ear. It also provides taste sensation to the anterior two-thirds of the tongue and sensory innervation to the nose and salivary glands.

This nerve enters the internal acoustic meatus and travels through the temporal bone. The facial nerve encounters its sensory ganglion, the *geniculate ganglion*, in the temporal bone. While in the temporal bone, the facial nerve gives off the following branches:

- *Greater petrosal nerve*—supplies efferent innervation to glands of the nose and mouth and the lacrimal gland (Figure 19-10)
- *Nerve to the stapedius muscle*—supplies the stapedius muscle of the inner ear
- *Chorda tympani nerve*—joins with the lingual nerve and carries taste fibers to the anterior two-thirds of the tongue (Figure 19-10)

The facial nerve then exits the skull through the stylomastoid foramen and gives off the following branches:

- *Posterior auricular nerve*—supplies the posterior auricular and occipital muscles
- *Digastric nerve*—provides innervation to the posterior belly of the digastric muscle
- *Stylohyoid nerve*—innervates the stylohyoid muscle

The facial nerve then enters the parotid gland. It bifurcates into two divisions, a superior temporofacial and an inferior cervicofacial (Figure 19-11).

The temporofacial division gives rise to:

- *Temporal branches*—supply the anterior and superior auricular muscles, frontal muscle, corrugator muscle of the eyebrow, and the orbicularis oculi
- *Zygomatic branches*—also provide innervation to the orbicularis oculi
- *Buccal branches*—supply procerus, zygomatic, quadratus labii superioris, nasalis, buccinator, orbicularis oris, and risorius muscles

The *cervicofacial trunk* gives rise to:

- *Mandibular branch*—provides innervation to the muscles of the lower lip and chin
- *Cervical branch*—supplies the platysma muscle

TABLE 19-2　INNERVATION OF THE TEETH AND TISSUES

Nerve	Teeth	Tissues
Maxillary Arch		
Anterior superior alveolar	Centrals, laterals, cuspids	Facial gingiva and periodontal membrane of anterior teeth
Middle superior alveolar	First bicuspid Second bicuspid Mesial buccal root of first molar	Facial gingiva and periodontal membrane of bicuspid area
Posterior superior alveolar	First molar distal buccal and lingual roots Second molar Third molar	Facial gingiva and periodontal membrane of molar area
Nasopalatine		Anterior palatal mucosa tissues Palatal mucoperiosteum from cuspid to cuspid
Anterior palatine		Molar and bicuspid palatal mucosal tissues Palatal mucoperiosteum from posterior of molars to the cuspid area
Mandibular Arch		
Inferior alveolar (the lingual nerve is usually involved)	All mandibular teeth	Labial mucosa anterior of mental nerve including lower lip Anterior two-thirds of the tongue (lingual nerve) Floor of the mouth (lingual) Lingual mucosa of all teeth (lingual)
Incisive	Bicuspids, anterior teeth	Chin and lower lip anterior of mental foramen
Mental		Chin and lower lip anterior of mental foramen
Buccal		Buccal mucous membrane of the cheek and gingiva of molars
Lingual		Lingual mucosa of all teeth Anterior two-thirds surface of tongue Floor of the mouth

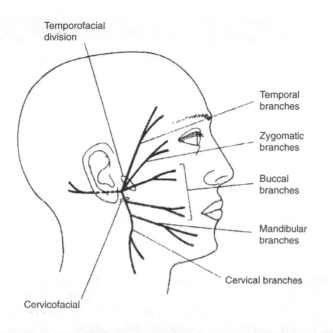

Temporofacial
division

Temporal
branches

Zygomatic
branches

Buccal
branches

Mandibular
branches

Cervical branches

Cervicofacial

FIGURE 19-11
Temporofacial and
corvicofacial divisions
of the facial nerve

THE GLOSSOPHARYNGEAL NERVE (IX)

The glossopharyngeal nerve is both afferent and efferent, and it exits the skull through the jugular foramen. Its branches are distributed to the tongue and pharynx. The branches of the glossopharyngeal nerve include:

- *Tympanic nerve*—provides parasympathetic innervation to the parotid gland and sensory innervation to the middle ear
- *Carotid sinus nerve*—supplies afferent innervation to the carotid sinus for its blood pressure regulators
- *Stylopharyngeal nerve*—supplies motor innervation to the stylopharyngeal muscle
- *Pharyngeal branches*—join with the spinal accessory (XI) and vagus (X) nerves to create the *pharyngeal plexus*. The plexus supplies the muscle of the soft palate and pharynx, except for the stylopharyngeal supplied by IX and the tensor veli palatini innervated by V. It also innervates the mucosa of the soft palate, pharynx, and tonsils. The glossopharyngeal nerve also supplies the posterior one-third of the tongue with taste sensation.

THE HYPOGLOSSAL NERVE (XII)

This nerve is the *motor supply of the tongue*. It exits the skull through the hypoglossal canal and is entirely efferent. It enters the mouth to supply the geniohyoid muscle and the intrinsic and extrinsic muscles of the tongue—with the exception of the palatoglossal muscle, which is innervated by the pharyngeal plexus. Damage to this nerve causes paralysis of the tongue. The tongue will deviate toward the affected side when protruded.

SUMMARY

The peripheral nervous system is made up of the nerves that travel *away from* the central nervous system; it *connects* all parts of the body with the central nervous system. There are 12 pairs of cranial nerves and 31 pairs of spinal nerves in the peripheral nervous system.

The cranial nerves provide innervation to the right and left side of the body, and they are usually designated by Roman numerals. The major cranial nerves include (1) the *trigeminal nerve*, which innervates the face, scalp, teeth, nose, mouth, and muscles of mastication and includes three branches—the ophthalmic nerve, the maxillary nerve, and the mandibular nerve; (2) the *facial nerve*, which innervates the muscles of facial expression and the muscles of the middle ear, provides sensory innervation to the tongue, nose, and salivary glands, and divides into eight branches—greater petrosal, nerve to stapedius muscle, chorda tympani, posterior auricular, digastric, stylohyoid, temporofacial, and cervicofacial; (3) the *glossopharyngeal nerve*, which supplies the posterior third of the tongue with taste and includes four branches—the tympanic, carotid sinus, stylopharyngeal, and pharyngeal; and (4) the *hypoglossal nerve*, which innervates the geniohyoid and the intrinsic and extrinsic muscles of the tongue.

WORKSHEET

A. Define the following terms.

sympathetic

parasympathetic

afferent

efferent

B. Complete the following chart.

Nerve	Sensory (S) Motor (N) Both (B)	Exit Function	Site
Trigeminal Ophthalmic (V$_1$) Maxillary (V$_2$) Mandibular (V$_3$)			
Facial			
Glossopharyngeal			
Hypoglossal			

C. Trace a pain impulse from the foramen rotundum to the maxillary right first molar.

D. Complete the following figure.

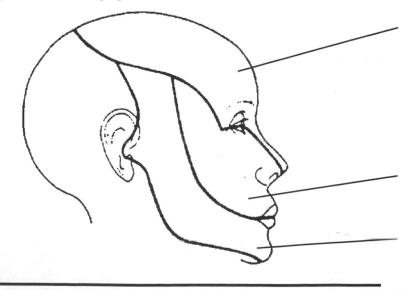

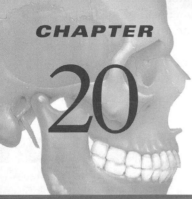

CHAPTER

20

Arteries of the Head and Neck

KEY TERMS

Artery

Vein

Internal Carotid Artery
External Carotid Artery
Veins of the Face

OBJECTIVES

- Describe the structures supplied by the internal carotid artery and branches of the external carotid artery.
- Describe the blood supply to the maxillary and mandibular teeth.
- Describe the structures drained by the superficial and deep veins.
- Complete the worksheet at the end of the chapter.

The head and neck are supplied almost entirely by the *common carotid arteries*. **Arteries** are tubes that carry oxygenated blood away from the heart. They expand and contract with the pumping beat of the heart. On the left side, the common carotid ascends from the *arch of the aorta*. On the right side, it arises from the *brachiocephalic artery*. The common carotid arteries are found on the lateral sides of the neck beneath the sternocleidomastoid muscle (Figure 20-1). At the thyroid cartilage, the common carotid artery bifurcates into the *internal and external carotid arteries* (Figure 20-2).

INTERNAL CAROTID ARTERY

This artery does not supply the mouth. It enters the skull through the carotid canal and supplies the brain and eyes. There are no branches present in the neck (Figure 20-2).

EXTERNAL CAROTID ARTERY

This artery ascends in the neck to the angle of the mandible. It ends as it is crossed by the posterior belly of the digastric and stylohyoid muscles. Its branches cross the face and scalp. The external carotid has eight branches (Figures 20-2 and 20-3).

1. *Ascending pharyngeal*: This artery arises just above the bifurcation of the common carotid artery. It travels on the side of the pharynx on its way to the skull. It supplies the pharynx and its muscles (Figure 20-3).
2. *Superior thyroid*: This artery also arises from the bifurcation of the common carotid artery. It supplies the thyroid gland and associated muscles (Figure 20-3).
3. *Lingual*: The lingual artery arises at the level of the hyoid bone. It passes deep to the hypoglossus muscle and enters the base of the tongue. The lingual artery ends at the tip of the tongue. It has three branches.
   a. *Sublingual artery*—supplies the floor of the mouth, sublingual gland, mylohyoid muscle, and lingual gingiva.

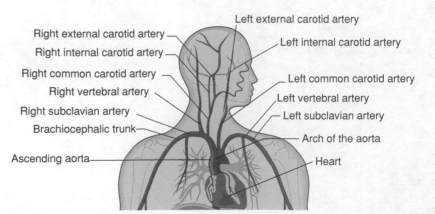

Right external carotid artery
Right internal carotid artery
Right common carotid artery
Right vertebral artery
Right subclavian artery
Brachiocephalic trunk
Ascending aorta

Left external carotid artery
Left internal carotid artery
Left common carotid artery
Left vertebral artery
Left subclavian artery
Arch of the aorta
Heart

FIGURE 20-1

Origin of the carotid and vertebral arteries

b. *Dorsal lingual artery*—supplies the back of the tongue, tonsils, soft palate, and epiglottis.
c. *Deep lingual artery*—supplies the tip of the tongue along its inferior surface (Figures 20-3 and 20-4).
4. *Facial*: This arises just below the angle of the mandible. It passes close to the posterior belly of the digastric and stylohyoid muscles, and enters the submandibular gland. It travels lateral to the inferior border of the mandible, and then it turns and passes in front of the masseter muscle. After crossing the mandible, it travels obliquely across the face to the eye (Figure 20-3). It gives off six branches:
a. *Ascending palatine artery*—supplies the soft palate, pharynx, pharyngeal muscles, and the tonsils. It arises at the beginning of the facial artery.
b. *Submental artery*—arises below the mandible and runs toward the chin. It supplies the sublingual and submandibular glands, mylohyoid muscle, and the anterior belly of the digastric muscle (Figure 20-5).

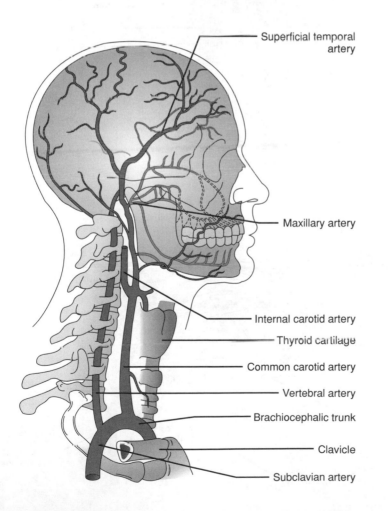

FIGURE 20-2
Course of the right common carotid artery

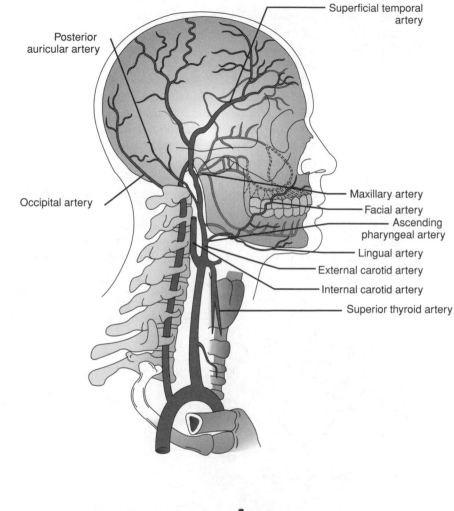

Posterior
auricular artery

Superficial temporal
artery

Occipital artery

Maxillary artery

Facial artery

Ascending
pharyngeal artery

Lingual artery

External carotid artery

Internal carotid artery

Superior thyroid artery

FIGURE 20-3
Branches of the external
carotid artery

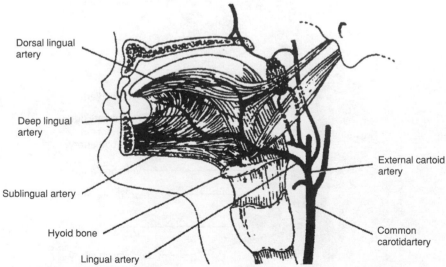

Dorsal lingual
artery

Deep lingual
artery

External cartoid
artery

Sublingual artery

Hyoid bone

Common
carotidartery

Lingual artery

FIGURE 20-4
Branches of the lingual artery

    c. *Inferior labial artery*—runs below the mouth, deep to the orbicularis oris, and supplies the lower lip and chin.

    d. *Superior labial artery*—runs above the mouth and supplies the upper lip. The inferior and superior labial arteries arise at the corners of the mouth (Figure 20-5).

    e. *Lateral nasal artery*—runs along the side of the nose and supplies the skin and muscles of the nose.

    f. *Angular artery*—the terminal branch of the facial artery. It supplies the eyelids and skin of the nose (Figure 20-5).

5. *Occipital*: This artery arises opposite the origin of the facial artery. It runs posteriorly toward the occipital area and supplies the scalp and associated muscles, the sternocleidomastoid, and the muscles of the neck (Figure 20-3).

6. *Posterior auricular*: The posterior auricular artery arises opposite the ear and travels behind the ear. It supplies the outer ear and associated scalp (Figure 20-3).

7. *Superficial temporal*: The superficial temporal artery and maxillary artery are the terminal branches of the external carotid artery. The superficial

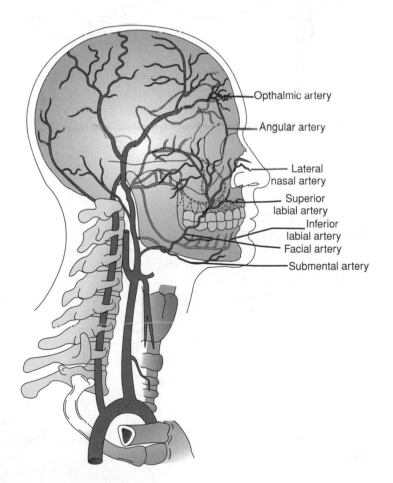

Opthalmic artery

Angular artery

Lateral nasal artery

Superior labial artery

Inferior labial artery

Facial artery

Submental artery

FIGURE 20-5
Branches of the facial artery

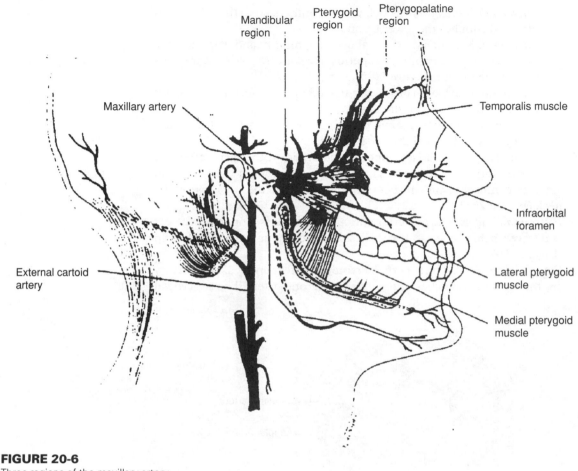

FIGURE 20-6
Three regions of the maxillary artery

temporal artery travels through the parotid gland in front of the ear. Before the superficial artery emerges from the parotid gland, it gives off the *transverse facial artery*, which supplies the masseter muscle and parotid gland. *Auricular* branches travel to the ear, and a *middle temporal* branch supplies the temporalis muscle (Figures 20-2 and 20-3).

8. *Maxillary*: The maxillary artery is the larger of the two terminal branches of the external carotid. It arises from the external carotid artery at the neck of the mandible. It passes between the mandible and spheno-mandibular ligament, close to the lateral pterygoid muscle, on its way to the pterygopalatine fossa. It supplies facial structures and is divided into three sections: *mandibular*, *pterygoid*, and *pterygopalatine* (Figure 20-6).

Mandibular Section

This section is located behind the neck of the mandible. There are five branches found here.

1. *Deep auricular artery*—supplies the temporomandibular joint, external acoustic meatus, and the tympanic membrane (Figure 20-7).
2. *Anterior tympanic artery*—supplies the inside of the tympanic membrane (Figure 20-7).
3. *Inferior alveolar artery*—travels with the inferior alveolar nerve and enters the mandibular foramen. This artery supplies the mandibular molar and premolar teeth (Figure 20-7).

   Before the inferior alveolar artery enters the mandibular foramen, it gives off a branch, the *mylohyoid artery*, which travels in the mylohyoid groove to supply the mylohyoid muscle. Also given off is a *lingual branch*, which aids in supplying the tongue. The inferior alveolar artery travels in the mandibular canal until it reaches the mental foramen, at which point it branches into the *mental artery* and *incisive artery*. The *mental artery* exits the mandibular canal through the mental foramen to supply the chin, while the *incisive artery* remains in the mandibular canal to supply the mandibular anterior teeth. Branches of the arteries enter the apical foramen to supply the pulp.
4. *Middle meningeal artery*—ascends between the lateral pterygoid muscle and the sphenomandibular ligament, and between the roots of the auriculotemporal nerve. It enters the cranium through the foramen spinosum to supply the dura mater and cranium (Figure 20-7).
5. *Accessory meningeal artery*—travels through the foramen ovale to supply the dura mater and trigeminal ganglion (Figure 20-7).

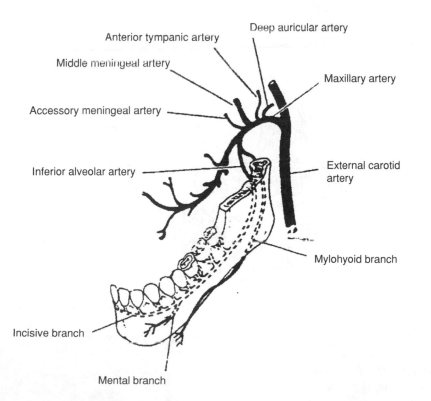

FIGURE 20-7
Branches of the mandibular section of the maxillary artery

Pterygoid Section

This section is located in the infratemporal fossa (Figure 20-6). It has six branches.

1. & 2. *Posterior and anterior deep temporal arteries*—supply the temporalis muscle.
   3. *Masseteric artery*—supplies the masseter muscle.
4. & 5. *Medial and lateral pterygoid arteries*—supply the medial and lateral pterygoid muscles.
   6. *Buccal artery*—supplies the buccinator muscle and the cheek.

Pterygopalatine Section

This section is located in the pterygopalatine fossa. The maxillary artery ends around the infraorbital area. There are six branches found here.

1. *Posterior superior alveolar artery*—travels across the maxilla with the posterior superior alveolar nerve. Branches supply the maxillary molar teeth, maxillary sinus, and associated gingiva (Figure 20-8).
2. *Infraorbital artery*—emerges onto the face through the infraorbital foramen. A *middle superior alveolar branch* supplies the maxillary premolar teeth. An *anterior superior branch* supplies the maxillary incisors and canine teeth. The lacrimal sacs and lower eyelids are supplied by the *palpebral branches. Labial branches* supply the upper lip, while *nasal branches* supply the nose (Figure 20-8).

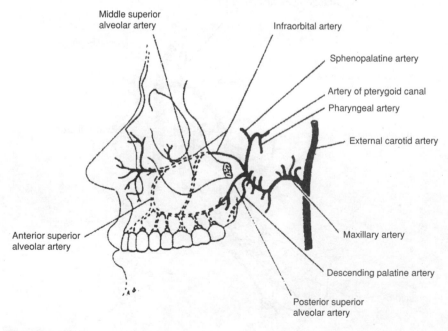

FIGURE 20-8
Branches of the pterygopalatine section of the maxillary artery

3. *Greater palatine artery*—emerges from the greater palatine foramen to supply the gingiva, palatine glands, and the roof of the mouth. The *lesser palatine branch* emerges from the lesser palatine foramen to supply the tonsils and soft palate (Figure 20-9).
4. *Artery of the pterygoid canal*—arises in the pterygopalatine fossa and enters the pterygoid canal. It supplies the upper part of the pharynx, auditory tube, and tympanic cavity (Figure 20-8).
5. *Pharyngeal artery*—runs posteriorly to supply the sphenoid sinus, upper part of the pharynx, and auditory tube (Figure 20-8).
6. *Sphenopalatine artery*—enters the nasal cavity through the sphenopalatine foramen. It divides into two branches (Figures 20-8 and 20-9).
   a. *Posterior lateral nasal artery*—aids in supplying the frontal, maxillary, ethmoid, and sphenoid sinuses.
   b. *Posterior septal artery*—supplies the nasal septum. One branch, the *nasopalatine artery*, travels to the incisive foramen where it joins with the greater palatine artery.

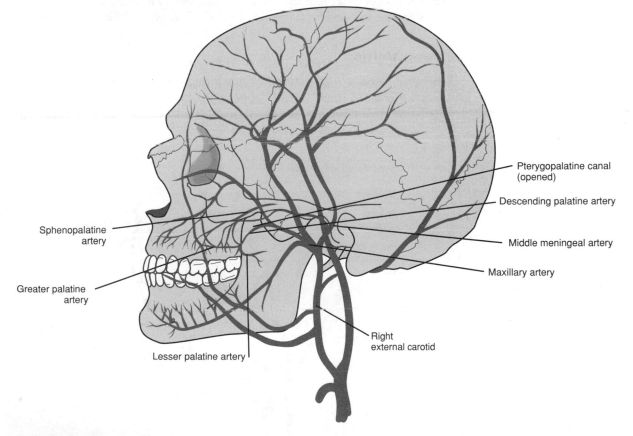

FIGURE 20-9
Greater palatine, lesser palatine, and sphenopalatine arteries

VEINS OF THE FACE

Veins return blood to the heart. Veins have valves that open in the direction of the flow of blood. The veins of the face usually travel with arteries and have similar names. Veins are commonly divided into a superficial and deep group. Variations in venous drainage are common. Facial veins do not have valves, so there is a potential danger of infection to the brain.

Superficial Veins

The *facial* and *superficial temporal* veins drain facial structures. The facial vein becomes the *angular* vein after it passes the upper lip. The facial vein has several branches from the nose, lips, eye, submental, and submandibular regions.

The superficial temporal vein joins the *maxillary* vein to form the *retromandibular* vein (Figure 20-9). This vein drains the regions of the maxillary and superficial temporal arteries.

The *common facial* vein is the union of the facial and retromandibular veins. It then enters the *internal jugular* vein (Figure 20-10). The internal jugular vein empties into the *brachiocephalic* vein. The right and left *brachiocephalic* veins join and form the *superior vena cava*, which drains into the heart.

Deep Veins

Pterygoid plexus is a collection of veins located between the temporalis and lateral pterygoid muscles and between the lateral and medial pterygoids. Structures that drain into the plexus include: muscles of mastication, bucci-

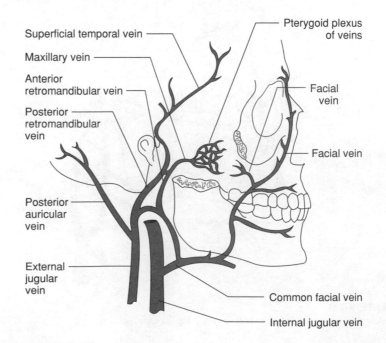

FIGURE 20-10
Internal and external jugular veins

nator, nose, palate, and the teeth. Injury to the pterygoid plexus during administration of local anesthesia can cause hematoma. The *maxillary* vein drains the pterygoid plexus (Figure 20-10).

SUMMARY

The head and neck are supplied almost entirely by the common carotid arteries. These are divided into three groups in the head and neck: (1) the *internal carotid artery*, which supplies the brain and eye; (2) the *external carotid artery*, which supplies the mouth and head and includes eight branches—ascending pharyngeal, superior thyroid, lingual, facial, occipital, posterior auricular, superficial temporal, and maxillary; and (3) the *veins of the face*, which generally travel with the arteries and are divided into superficial and deep veins.

WORKSHEET

A. Complete the following figures.

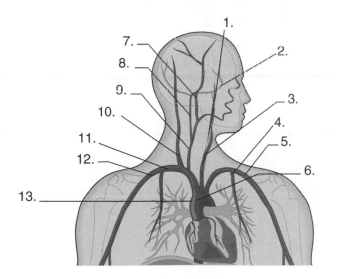

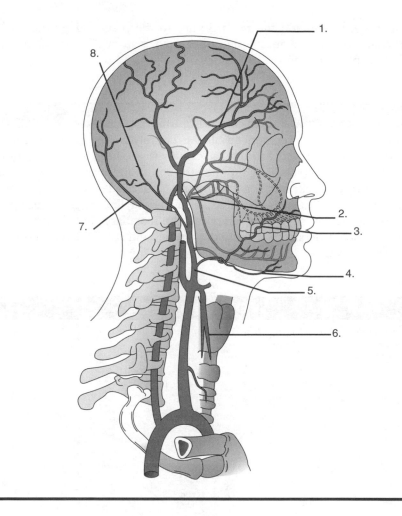

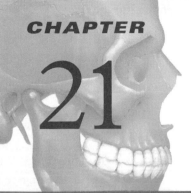

CHAPTER

21

Salivary Glands

Major Salivary Glands
Minor Salivary Glands

OBJECTIVES

- Differentiate between the major and minor salivary glands.
- Describe the location of the major and minor salivary glands.
- Identify the duct for each major salivary gland.
- Classify each of the major and minor salivary glands according to its secretion.
- Complete the worksheet at the end of the chapter.

In the oral cavity there are *major* and *minor* salivary glands. The three pairs of major salivary glands are the *parotid*, *submandibular*, and *sublingual*. Minor salivary glands may be located through the mouth.

MAJOR SALIVARY GLANDS

Parotid Gland

The parotid gland is the largest of the three major salivary glands. It is located on the side of the face, below and in front of the ear and behind the ramus. It terminates at the zygomatic arch in front of the ear and reaches down the masseter muscle. It extends inward to the pharyngeal wall. The duct for this gland is known as *Stensen's duct*, which crosses the masseter and buccinator muscles to enter the oral cavity opposite the maxillary second molar. Stensen's duct is covered by the *parotid papilla*, a small papilla extending from the cheek mucosa opposite the maxillary second molar (Figures 21-1 and 21-2).

The parotid gland is surrounded by a fibrous capsule. Several structures—such as the superficial temporal artery, the retromandibular vein, and the facial nerve—pierce the gland and travel within it. Saliva produced by the parotid gland is purely *serous*, a thin and watery secretion. The disease known as mumps is a viral infection of this gland.

Submandibular Gland

The submandibular gland is about the size of a walnut. It is located in the submandibular triangle, which is in front of and underneath the inferior

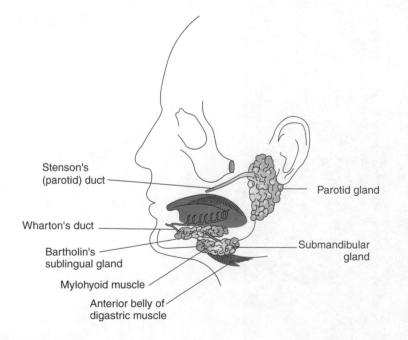

FIGURE 21-1

Locations and ducts of the major salivary glands

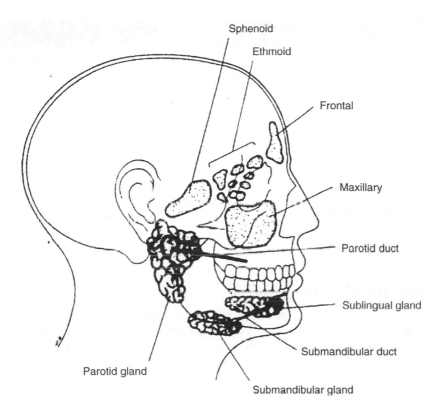

Sphenoid

Ethmoid

Frontal

Maxillary

Parotid duct

Sublingual gland

Submandibular duct

Submandibular gland

Parotid gland

FIGURE 21-2
Lateral view of the head showing salivary glands and paranasal sinuses

border of the mandible (Figures 21-1, 21-2, and 21-3). A small part extends to the mylohyoid muscle and lies deep to it. The remainder of the gland is located superficially to the mylohyoid muscle. The two divisions are connected. Its duct is known as *Wharton's duct*, which opens into the mouth at the sublingual caruncle.

A capsule encloses this gland. The facial artery is embedded in the submandibular gland. Saliva produced by this gland is mixed: 80% serous, 20% mucous. Mucous secretion is thick and viscous.

Sublingual Gland

The sublingual gland is the smallest of the major salivary glands. It is located beneath the sublingual mucosa in the floor of the mouth. This gland rests on the mylohyoid muscle, and its projection forms the *sublingual fold* or *plica sublingualis* along the floor of the mouth. It has several small ducts, 8 to 20 in number, known as the *ducts of Rivinus*. These small ducts empty onto the sublingual fold. It has one major duct, *Bartholin's duct*, which opens along with Wharton's duct at the sublingual caruncle (Figures 21-1, 21-2, and 21-3).

The sublingual gland is not encapsulated. It secretes a mixed saliva that is primarily a mucous secretion.

MINOR SALIVARY GLANDS

The minor salivary glands are small glands with short ducts that open directly into the mouth. Saliva secreted by these glands is usually mixed.

Labial Glands

These glands are found in the submucosa of the lips. They are numerous at the midline and have small ducts that open directly onto the lip mucosa. These are mixed glands, primarily mucous (Figure 21-4).

Buccal Glands

The buccal glands are located in the cheek. They are very similar to the labial glands.

Palatine Glands

These glands are found on the posterior third of the palate and on the soft palate. The opening of these ducts may be large and visible. They are purely mucous in secretion (Figure 21-5).

Lingual Glands

The lingual glands can be divided into three groups:

The *anterior lingual glands*, glands of the Blandin and Nuhn, are located at the apex of the tongue. The ducts empty onto the ventral surface of the tongue. They are mainly mucous in nature.

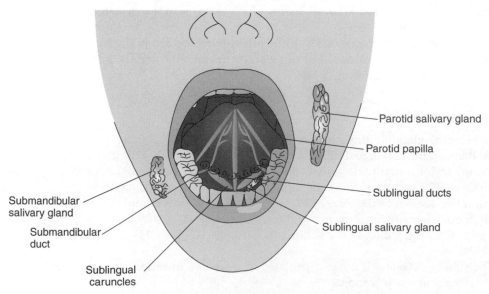

FIGURE 21-3
Major salivary glands and their ducts

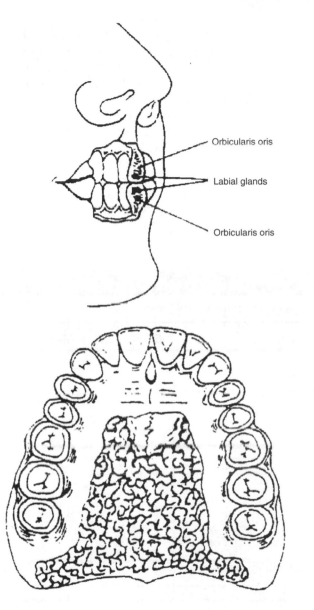

FIGURE 21-4
Labial glands

FIGURE 21-5
Palatine gland

The *lingual glands of Von Ebner* are found beneath the circumvallate papillae. Their ducts open into the trough of the papillae. They are purely serous.

The *posterior lingual glands* can be found near the lingual tonsils on the posterior third of the tongue. They are purely mucous.

SUMMARY

The oral cavity is supplied by major and minor salivary glands. The major salivary glands include (1) the *parotid*, which is located in front of the ear and supplies the mouth with serous saliva; (2) the *submandibular*, which is located in front of and underneath the mandible and supplies the mouth with mixed saliva; and (3) the *sublingual*, which is located beneath the sublingual mucosa in the floor of the mouth and supplies the mouth with mixed saliva, primarily mucous.

The minor salivary glands include (1) the *labial*, which are located in the lip submucosa and supply the mouth with saliva that is primarily mucous; (2) the *buccal*, which is located in the buccal mucosa and supplies the mouth with saliva that is primarily mucous; (3) the *palatine*, which is located in the lip submucosa and supplies the mouth with saliva that is purely mucous; and (4) the *lingual*, which are divided into three groups—the anterior lingual glands (Blandin and Nuhn), the lingual glands of Von Ebner, and the posterior lingual glands.

WORKSHEET

A. Place a check under the correct response.

Salivary Gland	Serous	Mucous	Mixed
Parotid			
Submandibular			
Sublingual			
Labial			
Buccal			
Palatine			
Anterior Lingual			
Lingual glands of Von Ebner			
Posterior Lingual			

Temporo-mandibular Joint

Anatomy
Nerve and Blood Supply
Movement

OBJECTIVES

- Describe and locate the following structures: condyle, mandibular fossa, articular tubercle, articular eminence, articular disc, capsule, and retrodiscal pad.
- Describe the innervation and the vascular supply to the temporomandibular joint (TMJ).
- Describe the two movements of the TMJ.
- Describe the etiology of internal derangement, subluxation, temporomandibular disorder (TMD), and arthritis.
- Complete the worksheet at the end of the chapter.

ANATOMY

A **joint** is a joining together of two bones. The **temporomandibular joint (TMJ)** is the articulation between the temporal bone and the mandible. It is bilateral, and movement of the right and left sides are interrelated and function as a single unit.

The osteology of the temporomandibular joint was studied in Chapter 17. The anatomy of this joint is depicted in Figures 22-1 and 22-2. The *condyle* of the mandible articulates with the *mandibular (glenoid) fossa* of the temporal bone. The specific location is the posterior slope of the *articular tubercle* and the anterior portion of the mandibular (glenoid) fossa. The condyle does not fit into the center of the mandibular fossa but rests closer to the articular tubercle. The condyle and articular eminence do not actually touch; the **articular disc (meniscus)** rests between them. This disc is

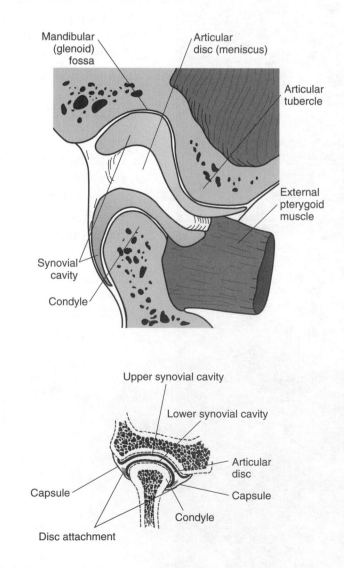

FIGURE 22-1
Temporomandibular joint

FIGURE 22-2
Temporomandibular joint

a pad of dense fibrous connective tissue that is thickest at the posterior ends, thinnest in the middle, and thicker again at the anterior ends. The articular disc, in effect, separates the temporomandibular joint into upper and lower joint spaces. Laterally and medially, the disc is attached to the condyle itself, so that whenever the condyle glides forward and backward, the disc moves with it.

The condyle and articular eminence are covered by dense collagenous connective tissue, which contains no blood vessels or nerves. **Synovial fluid** bathes these structures, providing nourishment and lubrication that enables the bones to glide over each other without friction.

A thick fibrous *capsule* surrounds and encloses the entire joint. The disc and capsule are fused anteriorly, and some fibers of the lateral pterygoid muscle insert into the disc. (Refer to Figures 18-3 and 18-4.) Posteriorly, the disc and capsule are not directly attached but are connected by means of a *retrodiscal pad*, a pad of loose connective tissue that allows for anterior movement of the joint.

NERVE AND BLOOD SUPPLY

Innervation is supplied by two nerves, the auriculotemporal and masseteric nerves, which are branches of the mandibular nerve (V_3). Blood supply is provided by branches of the superficial temporal and maxillary arteries.

MOVEMENT

Movement within the temporomandibular joint is essentially of two types: *hinge* (swinging) motion and *gliding* movement.

The hinge motion occurs in the lower joint space between the disc and condyle as the mouth opens. As the condyles begin this motion, the disc moves anteriorly with the condyles, because they are attached. As the mouth continues to open, the hinge motion also continues; but now there is an anterior gliding movement as well that takes place in the upper joint space between the disc and the temporal bone. The lateral pterygoid muscle (which inserts into the disc) causes the forward movement, and the condyle and disc move anteriorly until they reach the articular tubercle (Figure 22-3).

Closing of the mouth is accomplished by the lateral pterygoid muscle, which controls the posterior movement of the disc as well as its own contraction.

Clinical Considerations. An *internal derangement* occurs when the disc becomes stuck or displaced. As the condyle rotates and translates forward down the slope of the articular eminence, the disc should stay interposed between these bones. If it becomes displaced or stuck, sounds of clicking, popping, or **crepitus** (crunching) may result.

As the condition advances, catching or locking may occur. **Subluxation** takes place when the condyle is displaced anteriorly over the articular eminence and cannot be returned voluntarily to its normal position. As a result, the mouth cannot be closed, and prolonged spasmodic contraction of the muscles of mastication occurs. Subluxation can be corrected by wrapping the fingers in gauze and placing the thumbs on the occlusal surfaces of the mandibular posterior teeth. Then, by simultaneously pushing downward and guiding the mandible backward, the condyle can be returned to its normal position.

Temporomandibular disorder (TMD), characterized by muscle soreness, may occur with or without TMJ pathology or dysfunction. **Bruxism**, or grinding of the teeth, may be one cause of TMD, stress or tension may be another.

Inflammation of the joint—**arthritis**—may result from wear or tear within the joint or as a consequence of systemic disease such as rheumatoid arthritis. Cortisone may be used to alleviate the pain of arthritis.

SUMMARY

The temporomandibular joint is a complex, interrelated joint. Anatomic structures of the TMJ influence its function. The mandibular condyle rests in the mandibular fossa. The articular disc separates the TMJ into upper and lower joint spaces which perform either a hinge motion or a gliding movement. A capsule surrounds and encloses the entire joint. It is fused with the disc anteriorly; posteriorly, the disc and capsule are connected by the retrodiscal pad. Clinical concerns associated with the TMJ include internal derangement, subluxation, temporomandibular disorder (TMD), and arthritis.

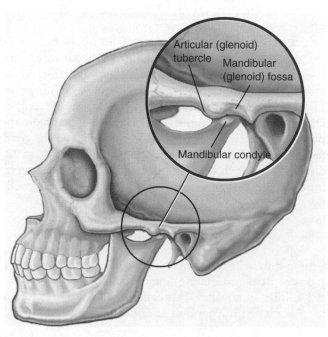

FIGURE 22-3
Temporomandibular joint

WORKSHEET

A. Answer the following questions and fill in the blanks.

1. What structure rests between the condyle and the articular eminence?

   _____

2. Describe the attachment between the condyle and the disc.

   _____

3. State the functions of synovial fluid.

   _____

4. Describe the anterior and posterior attachments of the capsule.

   _____

5. Briefly describe the two TMJ movements. When do they occur?

   _____

6. Describe the anatomical features associated with internal derangement, subluxation, and temporomandibular disorder (TMD).

   _____

   _____

7. Describe the nerve and blood supply to the TMJ.

   _____

Bibliography

Ash, Major. *Wheeler's Dental Anatomy, Physiology and Occlusion*. Philadelphia: Saunders, 1993.

Avery, James. *Essentials of Oral Histology and Embryology, A Clinical Approach*. St. Louis: Mosby, 1992.

Avery, James K. *Oral Development and Histology*, (2nd ed.). New York: Thieme Medical Publishers, 1994.

Bath-Balogh, Mary and Fehreback, Margaret J. *Illustrated Dental Embryology, Histology and Anatomy*. Philadelphia: Saunders, 1997.

Berkovitz, Barry K.B. and Moxham, Bernard. *Oral Anatomy, Histology, and Embryology*. Barcelona: Mosby-Wolfe, 1994.

Brand, Richard and Isselhard, Donald. *Anatomy of Orofacial Structures*. St. Louis: C.V. Mosby Co., 1994.

Carranza, Fermin. *Glickman's Clinical Periodontology*. Philadelphia: Saunders, 1990.

Fuller, James and Denehy, Gerald. *Concise Dental Anatomy and Morphology*. Chicago: Yearbook Medical Publishers, 1984.

Gray, Henry. *Anatomy of the Human Body*, (29th ed.). Edited by Charles Mayo Goss. Philadelphia: Lea and Febiger, 1987.

Hanson, Marvin L. and Barrett, Richard. *Fundamentals of Orofacial Miology*. Springfield, IL: C.C. Thomas Co., 1989.

Ibsen, O. and Phelen, J. *Oral Pathology for the Dental Hygienist*, (3rd ed.). Philadelphia: Saunders, 2000.

Jordan, R. and Abrams, L. *Kraus' Dental Anatomy and Occlusion*. St. Louis: Mosby Yearbook, 1992.

Massler, M. and Schour, J. *Atlas of the Mouth*. Chicago: American Dental Association, 1975.

McMinn, Robert M.H., Hutchings, Ralph T. and Logan, Bari M. *Color Atlas of Head and Neck Anatomy*, (2nd ed.). London: Mosby-Wolfe, 1994.

Melfi, Rudi. *Permar's Oral Embryology and Microscopic Anatomy*. Philadelphia: Williams and Wilkins, 1993.

Moss-Salentijn, L. and Hendricks-Klyvert, M. *Dental and Oral Tissues, An Introduction*. Philadelphia: Lea and Febiger, 1990.

Nield-Gehrig, Jill. *Fundamentals of Periodontal Instrumentation*, (4th ed.). Philadelphia: Lippincott, Williams and Wilkins, 2000.

Orban's Oral Histology and Embryology, (8th ed.). Edited by S.N. Bhaskar. St. Louis: C.V. Mosby Co., 1976.

Oregon State System. *Dental Anatomy, A Self-Instructional Program*. Norwalk, CT: Appleton-Century Crofts, 1982.

Phillips, Ralph W. and Moore, B. Keith. *Elements of Dental Materials for the Dental Hygienists and Dental Assistants*, (5th ed.). Philadelphia: Saunders, 1993.

Phinney, Donna J. and Halstead, Judy H. *Dental Assisting*. Clifton Park: Thomson Delmar Learning, 2000.

Ramfjord, S. and Ash, Major. *Occlusion*, (4th ed.). Philadelphia: Saunders, 1994.

Reed, Gretchen and Shepard, Vincent. *Basic Structures of the Head and Neck*. Philadelphia: Saunders, 1976.

Shapiro, H. *Maxillofacial Anatomy*. Philadelphia: Lippincott, 1954.

Wheeler, R. *An Atlas of Tooth Form*. Philadelphia: Saunders, 1984.

Wilkins, Esther M. *Clinical Practice of the Dental Hygienist*, (8th ed.). Baltimore: Williams and Wilkins, 1999.

Woelfel, Julian B., and Shcheid, Rickne. *Dental Anatomy—Its Relevance to Dentistry*, (5th ed.). Baltimore: Williams and Wilkins, 1997.

Appendices

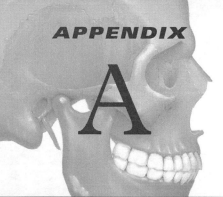

APPENDIX

A

Sequence of Tooth Development

TABLE A-1   PRIMARY DENTITION*

Deciduous Dentition	Formation of the Enamel Organ (Weeks in Utero)	Beginning of Calcification	Crown Completion	Average Eruption (Months, approx.)	Root Completion
MAXILLARY					
Central Incisor	10	3–4 mo in utero	4 mo	$7^{1}/_{2}$ mo	$1^{1}/_{2}$–2 yr
Lateral Incisor	12	$4^{1}/_{2}$ mo in utero	5 mo	8 mo	$1^{1}/_{2}$–2 yr
Canine	14	$5^{1}/_{4}$ mo in utero	9 mo	18 mo	$2^{1}/_{2}$–3 yr
First Molar	13–14	5 mo in utero	6 mo	14 mo	2–$2^{1}/_{2}$ yr
Second Molar	15–16	6 mo in utero	10–12 mo	24 mo	3 yr
MANDIBULAR					
Central Incisor	11	$4^{1}/_{2}$ mo in utero	4 mo	6 mo	$1^{1}/_{2}$–2 yr
Lateral Incisor	12	$4^{1}/_{2}$ mo in utero	$4^{1}/_{4}$ mo	7 mo	$1^{1}/_{2}$–2 yr
Canine	14	5 mo in utero	9 mo	16 mo	$2^{1}/_{2}$–3 yr
First Molar	13–14	5 mo in utero	6 mo	12–16 mo	2–$2^{1}/_{2}$ yr
Second Molar	15–16	6 mo in utero	10–12 mo	20–30 mo	3 yr

*From M. Ash, *Wheeler's Dental Anatomy, Physiology and Occlusion* (Philadelphia: W.B. Saunders, 1984).

TABLE A-2   PERMANENT DENTITION*

Deciduous Dentition	Formation of the Enamel Organ (Weeks in Utero)	Beginning of Calcification	Crown Completion (Years)	Average Eruption (Plus or Minus)	Root Completion
MAXILLARY					
Central Incisor	7	3–4 mo	4–5 yr	7–8 yr	10 yr
Lateral Incisor	7	10 mo	4–5 yr	8–9 yr	11 yr
Canine	7	4–5 mo	6–7 yr	11–12 yr	13–15 yr
First Premolar	7	$1\frac{1}{4}$–$1\frac{1}{2}$ yr	5–6 yr	10–11 yr	12–13 yr
Second Premolar	7	2–$2\frac{1}{4}$ yr	5–6 yr	11–12 yr	12–14 yr
First Molar	$5\frac{1}{2}$	At birth	$2\frac{1}{2}$–3 yr	6–7 yr	9–10 yr
Second Molar	6 mo after birth	$2\frac{1}{2}$–3 yr	7–8 yr	12–13 yr	14–16 yr
Third Molar	6 yr after birth	7–9 yr	12–16 yr	17–21 yr	18–25 yr
MANDIBULAR					
Central Incisor	7	3–4 mo	4–5 yr	6–7 yr	9 yr
Lateral Incisor	7	3–4 mo	4–5 yr	7–8 yr	10 yr
Canine	7	4–5 mo	6–7 yr	9–10 yr	12–14 yr
First Premolar	7	$1\frac{1}{4}$–2 yr	5–6 yr	10–12 yr	12–13 yr
Second Premolar	7	$2\frac{1}{4}$–$2\frac{1}{2}$ yr	6–7 yr	11–12 yr	13–14 yr
First Molar	$5\frac{1}{2}$	At birth	$2\frac{1}{2}$–3 yr	6–7 yr	9–10 yr
Second Molar	6 mo after birth	$2\frac{1}{2}$–3 yr	7–8 yr	11–13 yr	14–15 yr
Third Molar	6 yr after birth	8–10 yr	12–16 yr	17–21 yr	18–25 yr

*From M. Ash, *Wheeler's Dental Anatomy, Physiology and Occlusion* (Philadelphia: W.B. Saunders, 1984).

TABLE A-3 CHRONOLOGY OF THE HUMAN DENTITION*

PRIMARY DENTITION

	Beginning Calcification	Crown Completion	Eruption	Root Completion
Upper jaw				
Central incisor	3–4 mo in utero	4 mo	$7\frac{1}{2}$ mo	$1\frac{1}{2}$–2 yr
Lateral incisor	$4\frac{1}{2}$ mo in utero	5 mo	8 mo	$1\frac{1}{2}$–2 yr
Canine	$5\frac{1}{4}$ mo in utero	9 mo	16–20 mo	$2\frac{1}{2}$–3 yr
First molar	5 mo in utero	6 mo	12–16 mo	2–$2\frac{1}{2}$ yr
Second molar	6 mo in utero	10–12 mo	20–30 mo	3 yr
Lower jaw				
Central incisor	$4\frac{1}{2}$ mo in utero	4 mo	$6\frac{1}{2}$ mo	$1\frac{1}{2}$–2 yr
Lateral incisor	$4\frac{1}{2}$ mo in utero	$4\frac{1}{4}$ mo	7 mo	$1\frac{1}{2}$–2 yr
Canine	5 mo in utero	9 mo	16–20 mo	$2\frac{1}{2}$–3 yr
First molar	5 mo in utero	6 mo	12–16 mo	2–$2\frac{1}{2}$ yr
Second molar	6 mo in utero	10–12 mo	20–30 mo	3 yr

PERMANENT DENTITION

	Beginning Calcification	Crown Completion	Eruption	Root Completion
Upper jaw				
Central incisor	3–4 mo	4–5 yr	7–8 yr	10 yr
Lateral incisor	10 mo	4–5 yr	8–9 yr	11 yr
Canine	4–5 mo	6–7 yr	11–12 yr	13–15 yr
First premolar	$1\frac{1}{4}$–$1\frac{1}{2}$ yr	5–6 yr	10–11 yr	12–13 yr
Second premolar	2–$2\frac{1}{4}$ yr	6–7 yr	10–12 yr	12–14 yr
First molar	At birth	$2\frac{1}{2}$–3 yr	6–7 yr	9–10 yr
Second molar	$2\frac{1}{2}$–3 yr	7–8 yr	12–13 yr	14–16 yr
Third molar	7–9 yr	12–16 yr	17–21 yr	18–25 yr
Lower jaw				
Central incisor	3–4 mo	4–5 yr	6–7 yr	9 yr
Lateral incisor	3–4 mo	4–5 yr	7–8 yr	10 yr
Canine	4–5 mo	6–7 yr	9–10 yr	12–14 yr
First premolar	$1\frac{1}{4}$–2 yr	5–6 yr	10–12 yr	12–13 yr
Second premolar	$2\frac{1}{4}$–$2\frac{1}{2}$ yr	6–7 yr	11–12 yr	13–14 yr
First molar	At birth	$2\frac{1}{2}$–3 yr	6–7 yr	9–10 yr
Second molar	$2\frac{1}{2}$–3 yr	7–8 yr	11–13 yr	14–15 yr
Third molar	8–10 yr	12–16 yr	17–21 yr	18–25 yr

*Adapted from M. Ash, *Wheeler's Textbook of Dental Anatomy and Physiology* (Philadelphia: W.B. Saunders, 1992), 30.

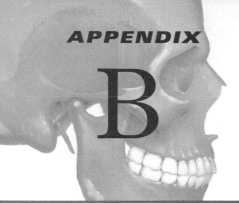

Measurements of the Teeth

B

MAXILLARY TEETH	LENGTH OF CROWN	LENGTH OF ROOT	MESIO-DISTAL DIAMETER OF CROWN	MESIO-DISTAL DIAMETER AT CERVIX	LABIO- OR BUCCO-LINGUAL DIAMETER	LABIO- OR BUCCO-LINGUAL DIAMETER AT CERVIX	CURVATURE OF CERVICAL LINE—MESIAL	CURVATURE OF CERVICAL LINE—DISTAL
Central Incisor	10.5	13.0	8.5	7.0	7.0	6.0	3.5	2.5
Lateral Incisor	9.0	13.0	6.5	5.0	6.0	5.0	3.0	2.0
Canine	10.0	17.0	7.5	5.5	8.0	7.0	2.5	1.5
1st Premolar	8.5	14.0	7.0	5.0	9.0	8.0	1.0	0.0
2d Premolar	8.5	14.0	7.0	5.0	9.0	8.0	1.0	0.0
First Molar	7.5	b1 12 13	10.0	8.0	11.0	10.0	1.0	0.0
Second Molar	7.0	b1 11 12	9.0	7.0	11.0	10.0	1.0	0.0
Third Molar	6.5	11.0	8.5	6.5	10.0	9.5	1.0	0.0

MAXILLARY TEETH	LENGTH OF CROWN	LENGTH OF ROOT	MESIO-DISTAL DIAM-ETER OF CROWN†	MESIO-DISTAL DIAM-ETER AT CERVIX	LABIO- OR BUCCO-LINGUAL DIAMETER	LABIO- OR BUCCO-LINGUAL DIAM-ETER AT CERVIX	CURVA-TURE OF CERVICAL LINE— MESIAL	CURVA-TURE OF CERVICAL LINE— DISTAL
Central Incisor	9.0†	12.5	5.0	3.5	6.0	5.3	3.0	2.0
Lateral Incisor	9.5†	14.0	5.5	4.0	6.5	5.8	3.0	2.0
Canine	11.0	16.0	7.0	5.5	7.5	7.0	2.5	1.0
1st Premolar	8.5	14.0	7.0	5.0	7.5	6.5	1.0	0.0
2d Premolar	8.0	14.5	7.0	5.0	8.0	7.0	1.0	0.0
First Molar	7.5	14.0	11.0	9.0	10.5	9.0	1.0	0.0
Second Molar	7.0	13.0	10.5	8.0	10.0	9.0	1.0	0.0
Third Molar	7.0	11.0	10.0	7.5	9.5	9.0	1.0	0.0

*From M. Ash, *Wheeler's Dental Anatomy, Physiology and Occlusion*, 7th Edition (W.B. Saunders, 1992). Reprinted by permission.
†In millimeters.

Directions for Drawing and Carving Teeth

DRAWING TEETH

1. Draw a base line representing the incisal and occlusal edge.
2. Measure the height of the crown and root; place a mark for each on the paper.
3. Draw a midline, for symmetry.
4. Divide the crown into thirds.
5. Place an "X" at the crest of curvatures.
6. Using the widest measurement, place the marks in the appropriate third. Be sure the midline is used.
7. Place "X's" in the cervical third at the narrowest points.
8. Connect the "X's" to conform with the shape of the crown as described in the reading.
9. Draw the root.
10. Draw specific anatomy as described in the reading. If the cingulum occupies one-third of the lingual, be sure that it is drawn in the appropriate space and with the correct curvatures.

Include other structures as fossae, ridges, and grooves.

CARVING OCCLUSAL SURFACES

1. Review the size and shape of the surface.
2. Review and draw the groove pattern.
3. Mark the location of the grooves on the waxed surface.
4. Carve an inclined plane toward the central groove.
5. Carve inclined planes toward the fossae.
6. Check the height of the triangular ridges and marginal ridges.
7. Recarve grooves.
8. Smooth and finish the surface.

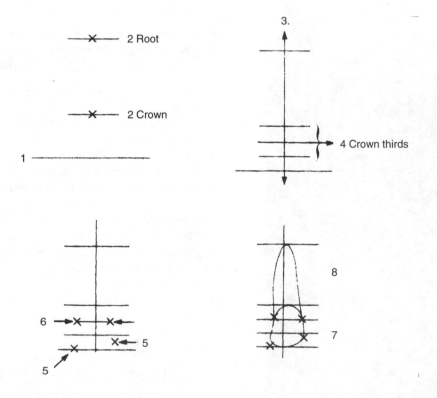

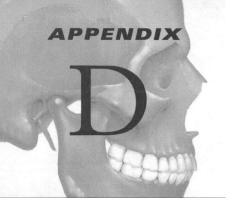

APPENDIX

D

Root Depressions and Cervical Lines

The chart on page 244 shows the variation of the cemento-enamel junction (cervical line), which curves occlusally from 3.5 mm on the maxillary central incisor to almost a straight line on the posterior teeth.

Also shown on this chart are the mesial and distal root flutings, or root depressions.

Familiarity with their location is essential to exploring and scaling the root surfaces.

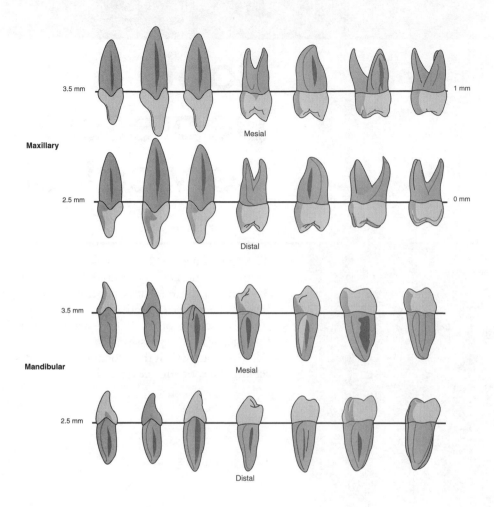

3.5 mm

1 mm

Mesial

Maxillary

2.5 mm

0 mm

Distal

3.5 mm

Mesial

Mandibular

2.5 mm

Distal

GLOSSARY

A

Abrasion—result of wearing away.

Active eruption—the emergence of the tooth from its position in the jaw to its position in occlusion.

Aesthetics—pertaining to appearance.

Afferent—nerves that carry sensory messages toward the brain.

Alignment—arranged in a row or a line.

Alveolar crest—the highest portion of alveolar bone.

Alveolar eminence—outline of the root on the facial portion of the bone.

Alveolar mucosa—thin, loosely attached mucosa covering the alveolar bone.

Alveolar process—that portion of the maxilla or mandible that surrounds the root of the teeth.

Alveolus—a socket in the bone in which the tooth sits.

Anatomic crown—the portion of the tooth that is covered with enamel.

Anatomic root—the portion of the tooth that is covered with cementum.

Angle's classification of occlusion—the first system developed to classify malocclusion.

Anomaly—a deviation from the normal.

Antagonist—a structure that opposes or counteracts another structure; in the oral cavity, the teeth that meet those in the opposite jaw.

Anterior—situated in front of.

Anterior tonsillar pillar—folds of tissue that extend horizontally from the uvula to the base of the tongue.

Apex—a pointed extremity of a structure.

Apical foramen—an aperture in the apex of the root.

Apposition—laying down of, or addition of.

Arch—a curvature; both the maxillary and mandibular teeth are positioned in an arch formation.

Artery—carries oxygenated blood away from the heart.

Arthritis—inflammation of the joints.

Articular disc—a pad of dense fibrous connective tissue that rests between the condyle and articular eminence.

Attached gingiva—the portion of the gingiva that can be observed on the external surface.

Attrition—wearing away by normal use (chewing, biting, etc.).

Autonomic nervous system—regulates functions over which we have no conscious control.

Axon—the process that carries impulses away from the cell body.

B

Bifurcated—divided in two.

Bifurcation—having two branches; forking into two parts.

Bilateral—both sides.

Bilaterally symmetric—the same on both sides.

Bruxism—grinding of the teeth.

Buccal—relating to the cheek.

Buccal ridge—a prominent feature in premolars that is formed by a well-developed buccal lobe.

Buccoversion—see Labioversion.

C

Calcification—process of hardening by the deposit of calcium salts.

Canal—a large opening through a bone.

Capsule—surrounds and encloses the entire temporomandibular joint.

Cementum—tissue that covers the root of the tooth.

Central nervous system—the brain and spinal cord.

Central pit—a deep depression where grooves merge.

Centric occlusion—the relationship of the occlusal surfaces of one arch to those in the opposing arch at physical rest position.

Centric relation—the relationship of the maxillary arch to the mandibular arch when the condyle is in the most retruded position.

Cervical—relating to the cervix or neck of the tooth.

Cervical line—where the anatomic crown and root join together.

Cervical ridge—a linear elevation of enamel from the cervix of the tooth.

Cervix—the neck of the tooth; the area where the crown joins the root or enamel joins the cementum.

Cingulum—an eminence or raised area on the lingual surface of the anterior teeth resulting from the lingual lobe formation.

Circumvallate—the largest of the papillae.

Clinical crown—that portion of the tooth visible in the mouth; it extends from the occlusal or incisal edge to the crest of the free gingiva.

Col—a "V"-shaped depression in the facial-lingual interdental papilla located cervically to the contact area of the tooth.

Comminution—pulverization, crushing, or grinding to a powder.

Compensating curvatures—curvatures of the arches that account for strength and efficiency in mastication and assist in the stability of the teeth.

Concave—curving inward; a depression.

Contact area—that portion of the proximal surface of a tooth that touches the adjacent tooth.

Convex—curving outward.

Cornerstone—refers to canine teeth, and their location at the corner of each arch.

Crepitus—crunching of bones in the temporomandibular joint.

Crest—a prominence or ridge; the height.

Crossbite—a facially positioned mandibular tooth or teeth.

Crown—the portion of the tooth normally visible in the mouth and covered with enamel.

Cusp—an elevation on the crown of the tooth.

Cusp of Carabelli—the fifth cusp of the maxillary first molar.

Cusp slope—the area extending from the tip of the cusp to both the mesial and distal contact areas.

Cuspids—refers to the maxillary and mandibular canines, which have sharp, pointed cusps.

D

Deciduous (teeth)—teeth that exfoliate or shed.

Deglutition—swallowing.

Dendrite—the process that conducts impulses toward the cell body.

Dentin—makes up the major portion of both the crown and the root of the tooth.

Dentition—arrangement of the teeth in the dental arch.

Developmental depression—a concavity in a surface that formed while the tooth was developing.

Diphyodont—having successive sets of teeth.

Distal—(the surface of the tooth) farthest from the midline.

Distal cusp—an elevation on the crown surface farthest from the midline.

Divergent—spread.

E

Ectoderm—the outermost layer of an embryo which will form the outer covering of the body and the lining of the oral cavity.

Edentulous—having no teeth.

Edge-to-edge—a contacting of the incisal edges or cusp tips rather than an interdigitation of cusp and fossae.

Efferent—the nerves that carry motor messages away from the brain.

Embrasure—a curvature on the tooth that allows the food to spill away (spillway).

Eminence—a prominence.

Enamel—hard tissue that covers the crown of the tooth.

End-to-end—see Edge-to-edge.

Endoderm—the innermost embryo layer that develops into the lining of the internal organs.

Eruption—the moving of the tooth occlusally.

Exfoliate—to shed.

External—on the outer surface.

F

Facial—toward the face.

Filiform—long, thin, more flexible papillae, that are grayish in color.

Fissure—a faulty groove.

Flared (divergent) roots—roots of posterior teeth that allow for growth of the permanent teeth forming beneath them.

Foliate—large raised papillae located on the lateral surfaces of the posterior third of the tongue.

Foramen—an opening in a bone or hard tissue.

Foramen caecum—a "V"-shaped terminal sulcus at the posterior area of the median sulcus.

Fordyce granules—small, yellow spots on the buccal mucosa and inner lip.

Fornex—vault or arch shaped.

Fossa—a shallow depression.

Fovea palatinus—two small indentations, one on either side of the raphe, located at the junction of the hard and soft palate.

Free gingiva—tissue attached only at the gingival groove that surrounds the teeth.

Free gingival junction—a slight demarcation about 1.2 to 1.8 mm from the gingival crest where the attached gingiva and the free gingiva merge.

Frenum—a fold of mucous membrane that connects two parts.

Fungiform—broad, round, red toadstool-shaped papillae.

Furcation—an area where the root trunk forks or divides.

Furrow—a groove.

G

Gingiva—the mucosa that covers the alveolar bone and surrounds the teeth.

Gingival crest—the prominent edge of occlusal or incisal gingiva.

Groove—a long, narrow depression.

H

Hard palate—the bony anterior two-thirds of the palate that is covered with mucosa.

Heart-shaped—a characteristic of the maxillary third molar.

Heterodont—different types of teeth with the same dentition (incisors, canines, molars, etc.).

Histodifferentiation—development into a specialized tissue.

Histology—the study of tissues.

Homodont—only one type of tooth in the dentition (e.g., all molars).

I

Ideal occlusion—a complete harmonious relationship of the teeth as well as of other structures of the masticatory system.

Incisal—the biting surface of the anterior teeth.

Incisive papilla—a small, raised, rounded structure of soft tissue at the anterior midline of the hard palate.

Inferior—lower.

Infraversion—a tooth positioned above the plane of occlusion.

Initiation—the starting of tooth development.

Insertion—the movable end of a muscle.

Intercuspation (interdigitation)—interlocking; a cusp-to-fossa relationship of the maxillary teeth to the mandibular teeth.

Internal—within.

Interproximal—the space between two adjoining surfaces.

Invagination—to enclose within.

J

Joint—a joining together of two bones.

K

Keystone—the mandibular first molar: its positioning in the arch is important for the appropriate alignment of the other permanent teeth.

L

Labial—relating to the lip.

Labial commissure—the closure line of the lips.

Labial ridge—a centrally located, well-developed middle lobe that extends from the cervix to the tip of the cusp of the maxillary canine.

Labial tubercle—a small projection in the middle of the upper lip.

Labiomental groove—a shallow linear depression between the center of the lower lip and the chin.

Labioversion—a tooth positioned more facially than normal.

Lamina dura—membrane covering or lining of tooth area.

Lateral—to the side.

Line angle—an angle formed by the joining of two surfaces.

Linea alba—a raised, white horizontal extension of soft tissue along the buccal mucosa at the occlusal line.

Lingual—relating to the tongue.

Lingual fossae—shallow depressions in the lingual surface of the tooth.

Lingual frenum—an elevated fold of soft tissue located on the floor of the mouth at the midline.

Lingual ridge—divides the lingual fossae into two segments.

Linguoversion—a tooth positioned more lingually than normal.

Lobe—a major center of tooth formation.

M

Major groove pattern—the deep grooves located on the occlusal surface of posterior teeth.

Malalignment—see Malocclusion.

Malocclusion—any deviation from the ideal positioning of the teeth.

Mamelon—a rounded prominence on the incisal edge of newly erupted incisors that are remnants of lobe formation.

Mandibular—relating to the lower jaw or mandible.

Mandibular torus—an overgrowth of bone occurring bilaterally on the internal borders of the mandible.

Marginal ridge—a linear elevation located around the perimeter of a surface.

Mastication—chewing.

Masticatory system—teeth and surrounding structures: jaws, temporomandibular joint, muscles, lips, tongue, and related nerves and blood vessels.

Matrix—a basic substance from which something forms.

Maxillary—relating to the upper jaw or maxilla.

Maxillary tuberosity—a small, rounded extension of bone, covered with soft tissue, posterior to the last maxillary tooth.

Medial—near the middle or medial plane.

Median sulcus—a shallow groove extending along the midline of the tongue, ending in a slight depression.

Melanin—a dark pigment.

Mental—relating to the chin.

Mesial—toward the middle.

Mesial concavity—a depression located on both the enamel and cementum.

Mesial interradicular groove—a deep groove located on the root of the maxillary first premolar.

Mesiolingual groove—in the mandibular first premolar, the groove that delineates the lingual cusp.

Mesoderm—the middle layer of an embryo which will form the skeletal and muscular systems, as well as the cementum, dentin, and pulp of the tooth.

Mesognathic—describes the normal profile.

Mixed dentition—presence of deciduous and permanent teeth in the mouth at the same time.

Modiolus—an area of intertwining muscles.

Morphodifferentiation—development into specific form or structure.

Morphology—the study of form or structure.

Mucogingival junction—the line of demarcation between the attached gingiva and the alveolar mucosa.

Mucosa—mucous membrane.

Mucous—thick, viscous saliva.

N

Nasal—relating to the nose.

Naso-labial groove—a shallow depression extending from the corner of the nose to the corner of the lips.

Neurocranium—the portion of the cranium that houses and protects the brain.

Neuron—a nerve cell.

Nonfunctioning cusp—a cusp that plays no part in occlusion.

Normal occlusion—conforms closely to an ideal occlusal relationship but involves some variations from it.

O

Oblique ridge—a linear elevation that transverses a surface.

Occlude—to close the teeth together.

Occlusal—relating to the biting surface.

Occlusion—the relationship of the maxillary and mandibular arch in a closed position.

Openbite—an existing space between the mandibular and maxillary teeth.

Oral cavity—the mouth.

Oral mucosa—the mucous membrane that lines the oral cavity.

Oral vestibule—the area between the inner lips and cheeks and the front surfaces of the teeth.

Origin—the fixed end of a muscle.

Overbite—a deep or vertical overlap of the maxillary teeth onto the mandibular teeth that exceeds the normal, or one-third the depth of the mandibular incisors.

Overjet—a horizontal overlap creating a protrusion or space between the labial surface of the mandibular incisors and the lingual surface of the maxillary incisors.

P

Palatine raphe—a junction of soft tissue extending vertically along the entire midline of the hard palate.

Palatine rugae—paired transverse, palatine folds of soft tissue on the anterior portion of the hard palate.

Palatine torus—a bony prominence of varied size located at the midline of the hard palate.

Parasympathetic—the system that slows heart rate and respiration.

Passive eruption—the increased exposure of the tooth. As a person ages, the gingiva recedes so that the clinical crown is greater.

Periodontal ligament—surrounds the root of the tooth, supporting and suspending the tooth in the alveolus.

Periodontium—the structures that surround and support the teeth.

Peripheral nervous system—composed of the nerves that travel away from the central nervous system.

Permanent teeth—the teeth that replace the deciduous or primary teeth.

Philtrum—a shallow depression extending from the area below the middle of the nose to the center of the upper lip.

Pit—a pinpoint of depression.

Plica—a fold of tissue.

Point angle—the area on the tooth where three surfaces meet.

Polyphyodont—having several sets of teeth during a life span.

Posterior—toward the back.

Posterior tonsillar pillar—a set of arches of tissue set farther back in the throat than the anterior tonsillar pillar.

Prefunction eruption—see Active eruption.

Primate spacing—the normal spacing between primary anterior teeth.

Prognathic—when the mandible protrudes.

Proliferation—rapid reproduction.

Proximal—nearest the point of attachment; the mesial or distal surface of the tooth.

Proximal surface—the surface of the tooth adjacent to the next tooth; refers to the mesial and distal surfaces.

Pulp—the only soft tissue of the tooth.

Pulp canal—the portion of the pulp in the root of the tooth.

Pulp cavity—the entire space within the tooth that contains pulp tissue.

Pulp chamber—the portion of the pulp in the crown of the tooth.

Pulp horn—the portion of the pulp chamber that extends toward a cusp.

Q

Quadrant—a fourth (of the dentition).

R

Raphe—a union of soft tissue.

Resorb—to dissolve into the tissue.

Retrognathic—when the mandible retrudes.

Retromolar area—a triangular area of bone, covered with soft tissue, posterior to the last mandibular tooth.

Ridge—a linear elevation.

Root—portion of the tooth that is located in the bone and not normally visible.

Root depression—a shallow, linear concavity located on the root.

Root trunk—that portion of the root that is not bifurcated or trifurcated.

S

Serous—thin, watery saliva.

Socket—a cavity in the bone; see Alveolus.

Soft palate—the posterior third of the palate, made up of muscular fibers covered with mucosa.

Somatic—nerves that supply muscles.

Spillway—see Embrasure.

Stensen's papilla—a small, raised flap of soft tissue on the buccal mucosa opposite the maxillary molar.

Stomodeum—primitive mouth.

Sublingual caruncles—round, elevated sections of soft tissue on either side of the lingual frenum, directly behind the central incisors on the floor of the mouth.

Sublingual fold—an elevated fold of soft tissue extending, medially, along the floor of the mouth toward the tongue.

Subluxation—occurs when the condyle is displaced anteriorly over the articular eminence.

Submucosa—the layer of tissue under the mucous membrane.

Succedaneous—a tooth that replaces or succeeds another tooth.

Sulcus—a shallow depression.

Superior—higher or above.

Supernumerary—exceeding a fixed number.

Supplemental grooves—additional grooves present in maxillary and mandibular third molars.

Supraversion—a tooth positioned above the plane of occlusion.

Suture—a joining of two bones.

Symmetric—exact form of both sides of a dividing line.

Sympathetic—the system that functions in response to emergencies.

Synovial fluid—the lubricating fluid of the joints.

T

Taste buds—these are located in the papillae of the tongue and are stimulated when food is dissolved.

Temporomandibular joint—the articulation between the temporal bone and the mandible.

Terminal mesial step—the position of a vertical plane along the distal surfaces when the deciduous second molars are in Class I position.

Terminal plane—the distal surfaces of the maxillary and mandibular deciduous second molars that are on the same line or plane.

Tonsils—lymphatic tissue masses found in the fauces.

Torsoversion—a rotated tooth.

Transverse ridge—a linear elevation that crosses a surface (usually the occlusal surface).

Triangular fossae—structures of premolars that assist with the grinding of food.

Triangular ridge—a linear elevation that forms a triangle.

Trifurcation—forked or divided into three (roots).

Tubercle—a small, rounded projection.

Tuberosity—a large, rounded projection.

U

Underjet—in the anterior dentition, when the mandibular tooth is facial rather than lingual to the maxillary anterior teeth.

Universal—common to all purposes.

Uvula—a downward projection of the soft palate made up of connective tissue, muscles, and glands.

V

Vein—returns blood to the heart.

Vermilion—red.

Vermilion zone—the pink border of the lips.

Visceral—nerves that supply internal organs (viscera).

Viscerocranium—the part of the facial skeleton that gives us our appearance.

Y

Y-shaped groove pattern—a feature of the occlusal surface of the mandibular second promolar.

Index